Direct Oral Anticoagulants in Clinical Practice

Editor

JEAN MARIE CONNORS

HEMATOLOGY/ONCOLOGY CLINICS OF NORTH AMERICA

www.hemonc.theclinics.com

Consulting Editors
GEORGE P. CANELLOS
H. FRANKLIN BUNN

October 2016 • Volume 30 • Number 5

ELSEVIER

1600 John F. Kennedy Boulevard • Suite 1800 • Philadelphia, Pennsylvania, 19103-2899

http://www.theclinics.com

HEMATOLOGY/ONCOLOGY CLINICS OF NORTH AMERICA Volume 30, Number 5
October 2016 ISSN 0889-8588, ISBN 13: 978-0-323-46314-0

Editor: Jennifer Flynn-Briggs
Developmental Editor: Kristen Helm

Hematology/Oncology Clinics (ISSN 0889-8588) is published bimonthly by Elsevier Inc., 360 Park Avenue South, New York, NY 10010-1710. Months of issue are February, April, June, August, October, and December. Business and Editorial Offices: 1600 John F. Kennedy Blvd., Ste. 1800, Philadelphia, PA 19103–2899. Customer Service Office: 3251 Riverport Lane, Maryland Heights, MO 63043. Periodicals postage paid at New York, NY and at additional mailing offices. Subscription prices are $385.00 per year (domestic individuals), $707.00 per year (domestic institutions), $100.00 per year (domestic students/residents), $440.00 per year (Canadian individuals), $875.00 per year (Canadian institutions) $520.00 per year (international individuals), $875.00 per year (international institutions), and $255.00 per year (international and Canadian students/residents). International air speed delivery is included in all Clinics subscription prices. All prices are subject to change without notice. POSTMASTER: Send address changes to Hematology/Oncology Clinics of North America, Elsevier Health Sciences Division, Subscription Customer Service, 3251 Riverport Lane, Maryland Heights, MO 63043. Customer Service (orders, claims, online, change of address): Elsevier Health Sciences Division, Subscription **Customer Service, 3251 Riverport Lane, Maryland Heights, MO 63043. Tel: 1-800-654-2452 (U.S. and Canada); 314-447-8871 (outside U.S. and Canada). Fax: 314-447-8029. E-mail: journalscustomerservice-usa@elsevier.com (for print support); journalsonlinesupport-usa@elsevier.com (for online support).**

Reprints. For copies of 100 or more, of articles in this publication, please contact the Commercial Reprints Department, Elsevier Inc., 360 Park Avenue South, New York, New York 10010-1710; Tel.: 212-633-3874, Fax: 212-633-3820, E-mail: reprints@elsevier.com.

Hematology/Oncology Clinics of North America is covered in MEDLINE/PubMed (Index Medicus), EMBASE/ Excerpta Medica, and BIOSIS.

Contributors

CONSULTING EDITORS

GEORGE P. CANELLOS, MD
William Rosenberg Professor of Medicine, Department of Medical Oncology, Dana-Farber Cancer Institute, Boston, Massachusetts

H. FRANKLIN BUNN, MD
Professor of Medicine, Division of Hematology, Brigham and Women's Hospital, Harvard Medical School, Boston, Massachusetts

EDITOR

JEAN MARIE CONNORS, MD
Assistant Professor, Division of Hematology, Brigham and Women's Hospital, Harvard Medical School, Boston, Massachusetts

AUTHORS

WALTER AGENO, MD
Department of Clinical and Experimental Medicine, University of Insubria, Varese, Italy

JACK E. ANSELL, MD
Department of Medicine, Hofstra North Shore-LIJ School of Medicine, Hempstead, New York

BENJAMIN R. BELL, MD
Member of Thrombosis Canada; Lecturer, University of Toronto, Toronto, Ontario, Canada

ROBERT DANNEMILLER, PharmD
Department of Pharmacy Services, Brigham and Women's Hospital, Boston, Massachusetts

JAMES D. DOUKETIS, MD
President of Thrombosis Canada; Professor, Division of Hematology and Thromboembolism, Department of Medicine, McMaster University, Hamilton, Ontario, Canada

JOHN FANIKOS, RPh, MBA
Department of Pharmacy Services, Brigham and Women's Hospital, Boston, Massachusetts

DAVID GAILANI, MD
Department of Pathology, Microbiology and Immunology; Hematology/Oncology Division, Department of Medicine, Vanderbilt University, Nashville, Tennessee

DAVID A. GARCIA, MD
Professor, Division of Hematology, Department of Medicine, University of Washington Medical Center, University of Washington School of Medicine, Seattle, Washington

ROBERT P. GIUGLIANO, MD, SM
Associate Professor of Medicine, Harvard Medical School; Cardiovascular Division, TIMI Study Group, Brigham and Women's Hospital, Boston, Massachusetts

ROBERT I. HANDIN, MD
Senior Physician, Hematology Division, Brigham and Women's Hospital; Professor of Medicine, Harvard Medical School, Boston, Massachusetts

JON A. KIMBALL, MD
Department of Orthopaedic Surgery, Harbor-UCLA Medical Center, Torrance, California

BARBARA A. KONKLE, MD
Professor of Medicine/Hematology; Associate Chief Scientific Officer; Director, Hemostasis, Platelet Immunology, and Genomics Laboratory, Bloodworks Northwest, University of Washington School of Medicine, Seattle, Washington

LOUIS M. KWONG, MD, FACS
Professor and Chairman, Department of Orthopaedic Surgery, Harbor-UCLA Medical Center, Torrance, California

ANG LI, MD
Senior Fellow, Division of Hematology, Department of Medicine, University of Washington Medical Center, University of Washington School of Medicine, Seattle, Washington

RENATO D. LOPES, MD, PhD
Professor, Division of Cardiology, Department of Medicine, Duke University Medical Center, Durham, North Carolina

ANNA PLITT, MD
Department of Internal Medicine, Mount Sinai Hospital, New York, New York

NICOLETTA RIVA, MD
Department of Clinical and Experimental Medicine, University of Insubria, Varese, Italy

CHRISTIAN T. RUFF, MD, MPH
Assistant Professor of Medicine, Harvard Medical School; Cardiovascular Division, TIMI Study Group, Brigham and Women's Hospital, Boston, Massachusetts

ALEX C. SPYROPOULOS, MD
System Director, Anticoagulation and Clinical Thrombosis Services, Northwell Health Systems at Lenox Hill Hospital; Professor of Medicine, Hofstra North Shore-LIJ School of Medicine, New York, New York

TUCKER WARD
PharmD Candidate, Department of Pharmacy Services, Brigham and Women's Hospital, Boston, Massachusetts

ALLISON P. WHEELER, MD, MSCI
Department of Pathology, Microbiology and Immunology; Department of Pediatrics, Vanderbilt University, Nashville, Tennessee

Contents

Preface: Direct Oral Anticoagulants in Clinical Practice   ix

Jean Marie Connors

The History of Antithrombotic Therapy: The Discovery of Heparin, the Vitamin K Antagonists, and the Utility of Aspirin   987

Robert I. Handin

> The administration of intravenous heparin to postoperative patients by Barritt and Jordan reduced the incidence of fatal and nonfatal pulmonary embolism and established heparin as the standard for parenteral anticoagulation. The coumarin family of vitamin K antagonists quickly became the standard for long-term oral anticoagulation. Aspirin became a widely used antithrombotic agent after the discovery that chronic oral administration reduced the incidence of secondary strokes and myocardial infarction. This article gives a brief history of antithrombotic therapy, including the discovery of heparin, the vitamin k antagonists, and the utility of aspirin.

Direct Oral Anticoagulants: Monitoring Anticoagulant Effect   995

Barbara A. Konkle

> In some clinical settings laboratory measurement of direct oral anticoagulants effect is helpful in guiding medical care, such as life-threatening bleeding, need for emergency surgery, renal impairment, severe hepatic failure, extremes of body weight, or in patients with bleeding or thrombosis on therapy. This article reviews approaches to laboratory testing to assess the anticoagulant effect of these drugs. Because of the wide variation in levels measured in patients on therapy and minimal clinical data from dose adjustment, dose adjustment based on levels is not currently advised. In addition, these drugs interfere with many clot-based laboratory tests and caution is advised in interpreting these tests in patients on direct oral anticoagulants.

Postorthopedic Surgery Joint Replacement Surgery Venous Thromboembolism Prophylaxis   1007

Louis M. Kwong and Jon A. Kimball

> Elective total hip or knee arthroplasty places patients at risk for venous thromboembolism (VTE). As our understanding of the pathophysiology of VTE after joint arthroplasty has increased, pharmacologic strategies have been developed to target different aspects of the coagulation cascade. Various approaches have been used as risk reduction strategies. In 2011 and 2014 the Food and Drug Administration approved rivaroxaban and apixaban as new oral antithrombotic agents. Although controversies remain with regard to the ideal VTE pharmacoprophylactic agent, this class of novel oral anticoagulants has been demonstrated to be safe and to be more effective than enoxaparin.

Non-Vitamin K Antagonist Oral Anticoagulants in Atrial Fibrillation   1019

Anna Plitt, Christian T. Ruff, and Robert P. Giugliano

For more than 50 years, vitamin K antagonists (VKAs) have been the standard of care for treatment of atrial fibrillation (AF). However, the numerous limitations of VKAs have led to the development of non-VKA oral anticoagulants (NOACs). There are 4 NOACs currently approved for prevention of thromboembolism in patients with nonvalvular AF. This article provides an overview of AF, summarizes basic properties of NOACs, and reviews the landmark trials. Current data on use of NOACs in special populations and specific clinical scenarios are also presented. Lastly, recommendations from experts on controversial topics of bleeding management and reversal are described.

Use of the Direct Oral Anticoagulants for the Treatment of Venous Thromboembolism   1035

Nicoletta Riva and Walter Ageno

In the past 2 decades, the direct oral anticoagulants (DOACs) have emerged as alternatives to the standard therapy (unfractionated or low-molecular-weight heparin followed by vitamin K antagonists [VKA]), for the acute and extended treatment of venous thromboembolism. The DOACs have a more favorable pharmacologic profile and a predictable anticoagulant response and, therefore, have the potential to overcome some of the limitations associated with the use of VKA. Several ongoing registries are evaluating the use of the DOACs in routine clinical practice and will provide additional information in less selected patient populations.

Use of Direct Oral Anticoagulants in Special Populations   1053

Ang Li, Renato D. Lopes, and David A. Garcia

Direct oral anticoagulants (DOACs) have been approved for the treatment of venous thromboembolism and atrial fibrillation based on randomized controlled trials (RCTs) of direct comparisons with vitamin K antagonists. Despite having more than 100,000 patients enrolled, safety and efficacy are debated in selected populations. Although DOACs are reviewed as a class of anticoagulant, pharmacokinetic differences exist such that different medications may be beneficial in distinct clinical settings. Synthesizing available evidence based on phase III RCTs, post hoc subgroup analyses, and pooled metaanalyses, this review provides an overview of DOACs and scrutinizes individual differences in their applications for the special populations.

Perioperative Management of the Direct Oral Anticoagulants: A Case-Based Review   1073

Benjamin R. Bell, Alex C. Spyropoulos, and James D. Douketis

The periprocedural management of patients on direct oral anticoagulants (DOACs) is a common but potentially challenging clinical problem because there are few prospective studies to guide clinical decisions. Retrospective analyses from randomized trials and observational data suggest that DOACs can be managed in a standardized manner, based on surgical and patient characteristics, that does not result in excess major bleeding or thrombosis. In a case-based manner, this article presents a perioperative DOAC management algorithm and reviews the available and emerging evidence supporting the safety and efficacy of this approach. A free online clinical guidance tool is available from Thrombosis Canada that includes the proposed management algorithm.

Reversal Agents for the Direct Oral Anticoagulants   1085

Jack E. Ansell

The vitamin K antagonists (VKAs) are associated with a significant rate of major and fatal bleeding complications. The new direct oral anticoagulants (DOACs), even though having a better bleeding profile than the VKAs, are still associated with serious bleeding. The anticoagulation induced by the VKAs can be reversed with both vitamin K and prothrombin complex concentrates, whereas the DOACs were developed without specific reversal agents. Although there is controversy around the necessity of a reversal agent, most clinicians agree that having a reversal agent for the DOACs would be beneficial. Three reversal agents are currently in development.

The Intrinsic Pathway of Coagulation as a Target for Antithrombotic Therapy   1099

Allison P. Wheeler and David Gailani

Plasma coagulation in the activated partial thromboplastin time assay is initiated by sequential activation of coagulation factors XII, XI, and IX. While this series of proteolytic reactions is not an accurate model for hemostasis in vivo, there is mounting evidence that factor XI and factor XII contribute to thrombosis, and that inhibiting them can produce an antithrombotic effect with a small effect on hemostasis. This article discusses the contributions of components of the intrinsic pathway to thrombosis in animal models and humans, and results of early clinical trials of drugs targeting factors IX, XI, and XII.

Regulatory Impact on Thrombosis Treatment, Prevention, and Anticoagulant Use   1115

Robert Dannemiller, Tucker Ward, and John Fanikos

Thromboembolism afflicts millions of patients annually in the United States and is associated with a significant cost burden. Oral anticoagulants provide clinicians with options for management of these diseases and their use continues to grow. Accordingly, regulatory, legislative, and nonprofit organizations have set performance standards with the goal of improving patient outcomes, ensuring patient safety, and reducing costs. Recent efforts in quality improvement have introduced changes surrounding regulatory requirements, surveillance, litigation, and oversight that clinicians should be familiar with. This article summarizes key updates related to the management of anticoagulant therapy as it relates to thrombosis prevention and treatment.

Index   1137

Direct Oral Anticoagulants in Clinical Practice

HEMATOLOGY/ONCOLOGY
CLINICS OF NORTH AMERICA

FORTHCOMING ISSUES

December 2016
Aggressive B- Cell Lymphoma
Laurie Sehn, *Editor*

February 2017
Lung Cancer
Roy S. Herbst and Daniel Morgensztern,
Editors

April 2017
T-Cell Lymphoma
Eric D. Jacobsen, *Editor*

RECENT ISSUES

August 2016
Imaging of Neurologic Complications in
Hematological Disorders
Sangam Kanekar, *Editor*

June 2016
Transfusion Medicine
Jeanne E. Hendrickson and
Christopher A. Tormey, *Editors*

April 2016
Global Hematology
Sir David J. Weatherall and
David J. Roberts, *Editors*

ISSUE OF RELATED INTEREST

Clinics in Laboratory Medicine, September 2014 (Vol. 34, No. 3)
Anticoagulants
Jerrold H. Levy, *Editor*
Available at: http://www.labmed.theclinics.com/

Emergency Medicine Clinics of North America, August 2014 (Vol. 32, No. 3)
Hematology/Oncology Emergencies
John C. Perkins and Jonathan E. Davis, *Editors*
Available at: http://www.emed.theclinics.com/

THE CLINICS ARE AVAILABLE ONLINE!
Access your subscription at:
www.theclinics.com

Preface

Direct Oral Anticoagulants in Clinical Practice

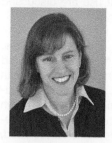

Jean Marie Connors, MD
Editor

Anticoagulant choices have increased exponentially in the last few years, with new options available for the prevention and treatment of thrombotic disease. Unlike heparin and warfarin, which were serendipitously discovered, these new anticoagulants were intentionally developed. Designed to target a single active coagulation factor, they bind to either thrombin or active Factor X to inhibit thrombus formation. While over twenty years elapsed from the time of discovery of heparin to its use in clinical applications, the direct oral anticoagulants (DOAC) rapidly became available for clinical practice. Results of the large phase 3 randomized clinical trials, which enrolled approximately 100,000 people, served as the basis for regulatory approval. Although these recently approved oral anticoagulants were developed for simplicity of use compared with warfarin and heparins—no need for monitoring plasma concentration, no dose variability from person to person, little drug-drug interactions—these medications are still anticoagulants with associated risk of bleeding. The practicing clinician should understand their major pharmacologic properties and be informed about how best to use these anticoagulants.

In this issue of *Hematology/Oncology Clinics of North America*, we briefly review the history of discovery of the first anticoagulants, heparin and warfarin, and their development for clinical use. We then focus on the DOACs and the information providers need to know for the effective and safe use of these agents in clinical practice. Experts in the field provide concise information on the currently approved indications for use, including postorthopedic joint replacement venous thromboembolism (VTE) prophylaxis, stroke prevention in atrial fibrillation, and the acute and extended treatment of VTE. Information on how to monitor the anticoagulant activity of these agents when necessary is provided. Expert opinion, incorporating the limited available data, is given on the use of these agents in the perioperative setting and in populations with characteristics that would have excluded them in large numbers from the major clinical studies, such as renal insufficiency, obesity, and age. Information about the reversal

Hematol Oncol Clin N Am 30 (2016) ix–x
http://dx.doi.org/10.1016/j.hoc.2016.07.015
0889-8588/16/© 2016 Published by Elsevier Inc.

hemonc.theclinics.com

agents for the DOACs is provided. The lack of reversal agents has been a major concern for both patients and clinicians and has been an obstacle for use for many patients. Lack of reversal agents should no longer be of concern as a specific reversal agent for dabigatran is now approved for use in the United States, Canada, and Europe, with the approval of a reversal agent for the Xa inhibitors expected by the time this issue of *Hematology/Oncology Clinics of North America* is printed. Finally, regulatory issues surrounding VTE treatment and anticoagulant use are discussed with their impact on clinical practice.

The anticoagulant field is evolving rapidly, and there is much to learn about these new drugs. Questions such as, should target levels be used for certain populations, what are those levels, and how do they vary by indication, all need to be explored and identified. These anticoagulants are not new any longer, and although novel in their direct targeting of specific activated anticoagulant factors, they are anticoagulants. Inhibition of thrombosis is also accompanied by impaired hemostasis, although to a lesser degree than with the traditional anticoagulants. Information on new strategies with different targets that might uncouple thrombosis and hemostasis is included, although these strategies are in the early phase of development and significantly more work is needed before they are adopted in clinical practice.

Although more information on DOACs will undoubtedly be available in the future, it will build on the basics that are included in this issue of *Hematology/Oncology Clinics of North America*. The authors and I hope that you will find this information useful and informative for clinical practice in the real world today.

Jean Marie Connors, MD
Division of Hematology
Brigham and Women's Hospital
Harvard Medical School
75 Francis Street
Mid-Campus 3
Boston, MA 02116, USA

E-mail address:
jconnors@partners.org

The History of Antithrombotic Therapy
The Discovery of Heparin, the Vitamin K Antagonists, and the Utility of Aspirin

Robert I. Handin, MD[a,b]

KEYWORDS

• Antithrombotic therapy • Heparin • Vitamin K antagonists • Aspirin

KEY POINTS

• The administration of intravenous heparin to a small number of postoperative patients by Barritt and Jordan dramatically reduced the incidence of fatal and nonfatal pulmonary embolism and established heparin as the gold standard for parenteral anticoagulation.

• The coumarin family of vitamin K antagonists quickly became the standard for long-term oral anticoagulation after 3 months of therapy dramatically reduced the recurrence of deep venous thrombosis in patients who had previously received a few weeks of intravenous heparin.

• Aspirin, which was a venerable antipyretic and antiinflammatory agent, became a widely used antithrombotic agent after the discovery that chronic oral administration reduced the incidence of secondary strokes and myocardial infarction by 25%.

Having practiced medicine for almost a half century, with a focus on coagulation disorders and antithrombotic therapy, I have become quite familiar with the classic antithrombotic drugs: heparin, warfarin, and aspirin. No one can dispute their effectiveness. The administration of intravenous heparin to a small number of postoperative patients by Barritt and Jordan[1] dramatically reduced the incidence of fatal and nonfatal pulmonary embolism and established heparin as the gold standard for parenteral anticoagulation. The coumarin family of vitamin K antagonists quickly became the standard for long-term oral anticoagulation after 3 months of therapy dramatically reduced the recurrence of deep venous thrombosis in patients who had previously received a few weeks of intravenous heparin. Aspirin, which was a venerable antipyretic and antiinflammatory agent, became a widely used antithrombotic agent after the discovery that chronic oral administration reduced the incidence of secondary strokes and myocardial infarction (MI) by 25%. Even modest doses, as low as 81 mg daily,

a Hematology Division, Brigham and Women's Hospital, 75 Francis St., Boston, MA 02115, USA;
b Harvard Medical School, Boston, MA 02115, USA
E-mail address: rhandin@partners.org

Hematol Oncol Clin N Am 30 (2016) 987–993
http://dx.doi.org/10.1016/j.hoc.2016.06.002
0889-8588/16/$ – see front matter © 2016 Elsevier Inc. All rights reserved.

permanently inhibit platelet cyclooxygenase and, thereby, for a few pennies a day, effectively reduce the recurrence of cerebral and coronary artery thrombosis and embolism.

Of course, no drug is perfect and each of these agents has a downside. One universal problem is that all of the antithrombotic agents marketed to date increase the risk of bleeding. Each of these drugs also has unique side effects. Unfractionated heparin is immunogenic and causes thrombocytopenia and platelet activation in 10% to 15% of recipients. The vitamin K antagonists require frequent laboratory monitoring to assess drug dosing and meticulous attention to dietary intake of vitamin K, as well as monitoring of interactions with other drugs that can either enhance or reduce anticoagulant activity. The management of patients taking a drug like warfarin is so complex that most large institutions have had to invest in a physician-supervised anticoagulant management service staffed by experienced nurses and pharmacists. They do so to enhance patient safety despite that insurers do not reimburse for this valuable service.

Aspirin is, perhaps, the easiest drug to administer, although there has been concern among cardiologists that some patients may be resistant to the agent. Most cases of resistance are due to noncompliance or to simultaneous ingestion of other nonsteroidal antiinflammatory drugs (NSAIDs), such as ibuprofen or sodium naproxen, which compete with aspirin and prevent it from irreversibly acetylating its most important target, platelet cyclooxygenase. A small number of patients do require more than the now standard antithrombotic dose of 81 mg per day and might be called resistant, at least to a baby aspirin. Doubling the dose usually overcomes the resistance.

What is remarkable about the discovery of heparin and the vitamin K antagonists, and the observation that aspirin has antithrombotic properties, is the serendipity and empiricism that led to these discoveries. Very little was known about the intricacies of blood coagulation or the genesis of thrombi when heparin and the vitamin K antagonists were discovered. The pursuit of aspirin as an antithrombotic involved a large leap of faith taken by a humble general practitioner. Moreover, by today's standards for drug development, neither the vitamin K antagonists nor heparin would garner Food and Drug Administration (FDA) approval, despite their long and illustrious histories as antithrombotic agents. As we enter a new era of antithrombotic therapy with modified heparin molecules, direct oral anticoagulants and the possibility, for the first time, of selective agents that may inhibit thrombus formation without increasing the risk of hemorrhage, it is worthwhile taking a look back to see how these 3 legacy antithrombotic agents were discovered and how they have been used to treat patients with thromboembolism because they provide the rock on which the exciting new therapies reviewed in this issue is built.

THE DISCOVERY OF HEPARIN: WHO DID WHAT WHEN?

Heparin is a highly sulfated, heterogeneous mixture of glycosaminoglycans of varying size and biologic activity extracted from animal tissues: liver, muscle, beef lung, and more recently, porcine intestinal mucosa. We now understand that heparin exerts its antithrombotic activity by binding to and enhancing the activity of the natural anticoagulant protein antithrombin 3. It functions in a catalytic manner, recycling from coagulation serine protease-antithrombin complexes to native antithrombin more than 30,000 times each second.

The discovery of heparin is a fascinating piece of medical history.[2] James McLean was an ambitious medical student from California who matriculated at Johns Hopkins with the goal of becoming an academic surgeon. In 1916, he obtained a position in the laboratory of Dr. William Howells, a pre-eminent Hopkins physiologist. He was assigned the task of purifying cephalin or thromboplastin, a tissue-derived or blood cell–derived phosphatide thought to initiate coagulation. His goal was to ascertain the purity of the laboratory's cephalin preparation, derived from dog liver, and confirm that its procoagulant activity resided in the purified phosphatide fraction and was not due to a contaminant. Unexpectedly, he found that certain phosphatide fractions separate from cephalin itself had anticoagulant properties. He published a paper on his finding in 1917 and demonstrated its anticoagulant property by injecting the heparphosphatide into living dogs.

McLean was awarded a fellowship to work at University of Pennsylvania in 1917 and did not continue work on the heparphosphatide there. He received a master's degree for his work on cephalin at Penn and was credited by Johns Hopkins for his second year of medical school. He then volunteered for the American Ambulance Corps and, in 1917, worked in France caring for wounded soldiers. In the fall of 1917, he returned to Johns Hopkins to finish his medical education. He also returned to Howell's laboratory but worked exclusively on cephalin, trying to develop ways to control surgical bleeding with cephalin-coated gauze. Howell, in his 1917 Harvey Lecture, credited McLean with the initial discovery of an anticoagulant phosphatide in liver. McLean had hoped to return to Howell's laboratory between his third of fourth year of medical school to resume work on the heparphosphatide, but this never materialized.

Another medical student, Emmett Holt, assisted Howell and isolated another compound from liver with anticoagulant properties, which they termed heparin to distinguish it from the heparphosphatide of McLean. Although McLean focused on cephalin and its applications, Howell continued to study anticoagulants from liver and, in 1922, presented a paper to the American Physiologic Society on the isolation of an anticoagulant molecule from an aqueous extract of liver, which did not contain phosphate but was rich in carbohydrate, particularly glucuronic acid. This material is most likely the compound we recognize today as heparin. The potential clinical importance of such an anticoagulant was quickly recognized and heparin attracted the attention of Nobel Laureate Charles Best and his colleagues at the Connaught Laboratories in Toronto. Best assembled a team of chemists, physiologists, and clinicians with the goal of establishing heparin as a useful drug. A Swedish group also began work on heparin with similar goals. By the 1940s, heparin was ready for clinical use. However, its debut was delayed until the end of the Second World War.

While the heparin project evolved in Canada and Sweden, McLean worked briefly at several academic institutions trying to establish himself as an academic physician. He eventually settled in Columbus Ohio in a private practice and worked in a local hospital. At this time, he initiated a long campaign to establish himself as the discoverer of heparin. He corresponded with Best and others on this subject and tried to argue that the material he isolated in 1916 was identical to the heparin later isolated by Holt and Howell, and further purified by Best and his colleagues. McLean wrote to many of the leaders of academic medicine and science about his role in the discovery of heparin and began a detailed account, which he never finished because of his death in 1957. Two years after his death, his unfinished commentary "The Discovery of Heparin" was published in *Circulation*.[3]

After the fact, it is hard to assess the 2 conflicting tales.[2] It is certain that McLean found something in dog liver that acted as an anticoagulant and I think he deserves credit for the concept of a natural anticoagulant. Howell and others are probably also correct that the material eventually developed into a clinically useful anticoagulant differed from the material McLean originally discovered in the Howell laboratory. Most people, who have not delved into all the details, believe McLean discovered heparin and did not receive appropriate credit. In fact, I have taught this to my students. I now think that McLean was over-reaching by demanding sole credit for the discovery. Had he been willing to share the credit with his mentor Howell and, perhaps, others in the laboratory who worked on the project, he might have died a happier man. We will never know.

THE DISCOVERY OF THE VITAMIN K ANTAGONISTS: SPOILED CLOVER, BLOODY CATTLE, AND RAT GENOCIDE

In the 1920s, in the midst of the Great Depression, cattle farmers began to notice that they were losing valuable livestock, cattle, and sheep, to a hemorrhagic disorder. Veterinarians and the farmers began to realize that the afflicted animals had eaten spoiled batches of a dietary staple, sweet clover.[4] The damp hay had become contaminated with penicillium molds. In the past, when sweet clover had spoiled, farmers bought supplemental feed. Given their economic straits, this was not possible during the Depression, so many animals perished.

A decade after the initial reports of sweet clover disease, Ed Carlson, a Wisconsin farmer, distraught over the loss of his cattle from internal hemorrhage and skeptical about the spoiled sweet clover theory of their demise, put a dead cow and a milk can of the cow's unclotted blood in the back of his pickup truck and drove 200 miles in a blizzard to the University of Wisconsin Agricultural Station where Karl Link and his student Wilhelm Schofield were working. He presented Link and Schofield with the milk can of blood and showed them his dead cow. Link had little to offer except advising Carlson to avoid feeding his cattle sweet clover and considering a transfusion of normal blood for afflicted cattle. However, he and Schofield did examine the blood and decided that it was time to try to purify the chemical in spoiled clover that had rendered the blood unable to coagulate. Six years later, Link and his colleagues had crystallized the substance: 3-3'-methylene-bis[4-hydroxycoumarin] in sweet clover. The precursor, coumarin itself, was harmless but became oxidized to this new compound with anticoagulant properties, later known as dicoumarol. The research had been funded by the Wisconsin Alumni Research Foundation (WARF), which obtained the patent rights for dicoumarol in 1941.

Although the discovery of dicoumarol solved the sweet clover mystery, there was no immediate use for the molecule. However, in 1945, Link had the idea to use a coumarin derivative as a rodenticide and began to look for a suitable compound that could rapidly and efficiently kill rats.[3,5] One compound, named warfarin, after the funding agency, WARF, was particularly effective and became commercially available. Subsequently, longer acting coumarin derivatives such as brodifacoum were developed and are widely used to control rodent populations.

Although a few forward thinking physicians, including Irving Wright at the New York Hospital/Cornell Medical Center, started giving patients with thrombophlebitis dicoumarol in the 1940s, many physicians were horrified at the idea of giving their patients rat poison, so the field languished. There was a big breakthrough in 1955 when President Dwight Eisenhower was hospitalized at Walter Reed Army Hospital with a MI and his doctors gave him warfarin. Treatment of this popular figure with rat poison seemed to remove much of the stigma, so that clinical application grew rapidly. The widespread use of warfarin required the development of better tests for laboratory monitoring and, eventually, sophisticated anticoagulant management services.

THE UTILITY OF ASPIRIN AS AN ANTITHROMBOTIC AGENT: A NEW USE FOR AN ANCIENT DRUG

The antipyretic and antiinflammatory properties of willow bark have been known since the days of Galen and Hippocrates.[6] Salicylic acid, derived from willow bark, was shown to be the active agent and became a popular medication in the nineteenth century. Salicylates were especially useful for the relief of pain and the treatment of patients with rheumatism. Although acetylsalicylic acid was first synthesized in 1853, Felix Hoffman, a German chemist working for Bayer, worked out the first large-scale synthetic procedure to add an acetyl group to salicylic acid in 1897. Acetylsalicylic acid, or aspirin, retained the antiinflammatory properties of willow bark and salicylic acid but was less irritating to the gastrointestinal tract. Although corporate executives were initially skeptical about its utility, aspirin eventually became a widely prescribed agent for relief of pain and inflammation. Literally, tons of aspirin are sold around the world annually.

In the 1940s, there was little understanding of the pathogenesis of MI. There had been some unsuccessful attempts to treat MI with the recently discovered vitamin K antagonist dicumarol. Despite pathologic findings of vessel occlusion and coronary thrombi, there were still doubts about the role of thrombosis in the pathogenesis of MI. Inexplicably, Dr Lawrence Craven, a general practitioner practicing in Glendale, California, a Los Angeles suburb, decided to test the hypothesis that aspirin might prevent MI. Dr Craven had no scientific or academic background. He had graduated from The University of Minnesota, served in World War I, and then settled in Glendale, working out of the Glendale Memorial Hospital.

Dr Craven devised an uncontrolled, nonrandomized experiment. He simply asked men in his practice between 45 and 65 who were overweight and lived sedentary lifestyles, which he reasoned increased their risk of having a MI, to take a daily aspirin. He observed that none of these patients had a MI during subsequent years of observation.[7–9] Although the experiment was deceptively simple, his rationale was sound and well-researched. He cited studies showing that high doses of aspirin prolonged the prothrombin time and noted that, in published studies and his own practice, patients who chewed aspirin gum after tonsillectomy had an increased frequency of bleeding, suggesting that aspirin had anticoagulant properties. He also noted that heart attacks were more common in men and attributed this to the more frequent use of aspirin for minor aches and pains by women. In fact, as he initiated his studies, some of his male patients were reluctant to take aspirin because it was "effeminate."

After his initial publication, he received correspondence from other physicians who had noted a similar beneficial effect from regular aspirin ingestion. He wrote of his experiments with restraint and humility, noting that the administration of aspirin was safe, did not contradict independent clinical findings, and that his findings were not arrived at with strict scientific methodology. I have not discussed these papers with any biostatisticians or modern clinical trialists to assess whether they were well designed and sufficiently powered to measure the observed effect, but it is impressive that he tested his hypothesis on a cohort of 8000 patients over many years. He had no assistants and no data managers, nor did he have to deal with complexities of institutional review boards or the FDA. Despite the prescience of the work and its importance to public health, his observations were published in obscure journals and received little attention. One wonders if he had attempted to publish the work in more widely read and more prestigious journals if it may have been rejected for lack of rigor. How many lives might have been saved if his empirical observation, perhaps strengthened by the endorsement of a major journal, had been widely adopted decades earlier?

The second part of the aspirin story is the unraveling of its unique effect on hemostasis, which occurred decades after Craven's observational trials had been completed.[6] Work on aspirin-sensitive signaling pathways, indirectly, led to the awarding of a Nobel Prize to the British pharmacologist Sir John Vane. Armand Quick, who invented the prothrombin time, observed that low doses of aspirin prolonged the bleeding time. Harvey Weiss, a New York hematologist then asked the important question: did aspirin inhibit platelet function? Indeed, he found that aspirin impaired adenosine diphosphate (ADP) release from platelets and ADP-induced secondary aggregation. He also noted that these inhibitory effects required the acetyl group present on aspirin because they were not induced by salicylic acid. He also observed that the antiplatelet effect of aspirin was rapid in onset and irreversible.

At about the same time as the seminal studies of Weiss, Priscilla Piper and Sir John Vane asked whether aspirin might inhibit prostaglandin synthesis. Vane had developed an elegant bioassay system to detect bioactive substances that induced or inhibited vessel contraction. He used this system to document that aspirin inhibited the production of all prostaglandins. With this system he also discovered 2 important new compounds: thromboxane A_2, a platelet-derived product that was a potent vasoconstrictor and platelet agonist; and prostaglandin I_2, or prostacyclin, a novel endothelial cell prostaglandin that was a vasodilator and platelet inhibitor. Vane received the Nobel Prize in 1982 for this important body of work.

This elegant basic science was advanced by a series of elegant clinical trials that established aspirin as an effective drug for the primary and secondary prevention of acute MI and strokes. These modern clinical trials confirmed and extended the pioneering observations of Craven. To illustrate how far we have come, aspirin is now immediately dispensed to any patient who arrives in an emergency room with chest pain, in case they are having an MI.

SUMMARY

Many years ago, I invited the late William Castle to deliver a talk on "The history of the discovery of vitamin B12 and its role in hematopoiesis" to the Boston Blood Club. Because most of the seminal work on this subject was carried out locally, much of it by Dr Castle, this seemed like a good topic. Always gracious, he accepted the invitation without hesitation. After the talk, which was very well received, he commented, "Bob, you know you are old when people ask you to discuss the history of a field rather than ongoing work." Compared with Dr. Castle, my contributions to the fields of hemostasis and antithrombotic therapy have been modest. I do hope, however, that this brief review provides some insight into the twists and turns and the unexpected contributors who helped to develop an important class of drugs. Who could have predicted that an astute general practitioner, an ambitious medical student, and a frustrated farmer with dying cattle could change the course of history and help to develop the first generation of effective antithrombotic drugs? I am sure there are stories to be told about the development of the new generation of antithrombotic agents discussed elsewhere in this issue; perhaps they will be even more entertaining.

REFERENCES

1. Barritt DW, Jordan SC. Clinical features of pulmonary embolism. Lancet 1961; 1(7180):729–32.

2. Marcum JA. The origin of the dispute over the discovery of heparin. J Hist Med Allied Sci 2000;55(1):37–66.

3. Wardrop D, Keeling D. The story of the discovery of heparin and warfarin. Br J Haematol 2008;141(6):757–63.
4. Duxbury BM, Poller L. The oral anticoagulant saga: past, present, and future. Clin Appl Thromb Hemost 2001;7(4):269–75.
5. Last JA. The missing link: the story of Karl Paul Link. Toxicol Sci 2002;66(1):4–6.
6. Miner J, Hoffhines A. The discovery of aspirin's antithrombotic effects. Tex Heart Inst J 2007;34(2):179–86.
7. Craven LL. Coronary thrombosis can be prevented. J Insur Med 1950;5(4):47–8.
8. Craven LL. Acetylsalicylic acid, possible preventive of coronary thrombosis. Ann West Med Surg 1950;4(2):95.
9. Craven LL. Prevention of coronary and cerebral thrombosis. Miss Valley Med J 1956;78(5):213–5.

Direct Oral Anticoagulants

Monitoring Anticoagulant Effect

Barbara A. Konkle, MD

KEYWORDS

- Oral anticoagulants • Coagulation testing • Trough level • Anticoagulant effect

KEY POINTS

- The direct oral anticoagulants (DOACs), dabigatran, apixaban, edoxaban, and rivaroxaban, were approved for prevention and treatment of venous thrombosis and for prevention of embolic stroke in patients with atrial fibrillation, without need to monitor drug activity levels.
- Clinical circumstances exist where laboratory measures of drug activity may help guide clinical care.
- Trough drug levels correlate best with bleeding risk, although values measured in patients on the medications vary widely.
- Screening laboratory tests differ in their sensitivity to the drugs and knowledge of the assays available and laboratory-specific performance is required.
- Direct oral anticoagulants can affect clot-based coagulation assays performed, including tests for thrombophilias, factor levels, and thromboelastography, and results of those tests should be interpreted with caution in patients on DOACs.

INTRODUCTION

Direct oral anticoagulants (DOACs) inhibit coagulation through factor Xa (apixaban, edoxaban, rivaroxaban) or thrombin (dabigatran) (**Fig. 1**), and do not require antithrombin for activity as is needed for the heparins and fondaparinux. DOACs are approved for prevention and treatment of venous thromboembolism and for treatment of patients with atrial fibrillation. Clinical trials were designed and regulatory approval given without a need for dose adjustment based on laboratory testing. In clinical trials use of these agents was associated with less or similar bleeding and thrombotic complications compared with warfarin.[1–8] However, in certain clinical settings measurement of anticoagulant activity is desired to help inform patient care. These include life-threatening bleeding, emergency surgery, renal impairment, liver failure, in patients taking medications that affect DOAC plasma concentrations, recurrent thrombosis or bleeding on recommended doses, or extremes of body weight (**Box 1**).

Disclosure: The author has nothing to disclose.
Clinical and Translational Research, Hemostasis, Platelet Immunology, and Genomics Laboratory, Bloodworks Northwest, University of Washington School of Medicine, 921 Terry Avenue, Seattle, WA 98104, USA
E-mail address: BarbaraK@BloodworksNW.org

Hematol Oncol Clin N Am 30 (2016) 995–1006
http://dx.doi.org/10.1016/j.hoc.2016.05.004
0889-8588/16/© 2016 Elsevier Inc. All rights reserved.
hemonc.theclinics.com

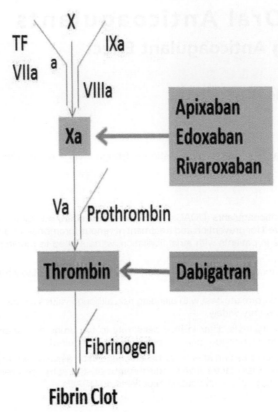

Fig. 1. Sites of action of DOACs. TF, tissue factor. [a] This activation pathway is inhibited on formation of an Xa-tissue factor pathway inhibitor-VIIa-TF complex.

True therapeutic ranges based on clinical outcomes have not been established for these agents. Levels that correlate with efficacy and/or adverse outcomes are just now being studied. Instead we have levels that were measured in study populations on standard dosing, most commonly at peak and trough concentrations using liquid chromatography/tandem mass spectrometry (LC-MS/MS) methodology. Of note, these levels vary widely across study participants.[9–12] Instead of therapeutic levels, the terms on-therapy drug concentrations or on-therapy levels are more accurate.

Box 1
Reasons for measuring DOAC anticoagulant activity
Major bleeding
Emergent need for surgery
Renal impairment
Severe liver failure
Potential drug-drug interactions
Bleeding or thrombosis on therapy
Extremes of body weight

The pharmacology of the DOACs is discussed in detail elsewhere (see Robert I. Handin's article, "The History of Antithrombotic Therapy — The Discovery of Heparin, the Vitamin K Antagonists and the Utility of Aspirin," in this issue). Overall the drugs are similar in peak levels (1–4 hours) and half-life (approximately 7–12 hours). The latter depends, in part, on age and comorbid conditions. Additional key drug characteristics when considering laboratory monitoring are shown in **Table 1**.

DIAGNOSTIC OPTIONS
Direct Oral Anticoagulants and Coagulation Testing

Although clinicians may consider measurement of DOAC-induced anticoagulant activity in several settings, they should be cautioned before testing clinically stable patients, given the wide range of on-therapy drug concentrations that have been measured in subjects receiving standard dosing. Also, given the relatively short half-life of these drugs, the levels are not a measure of drug adherence as the international normalized ratio (INR) is for warfarin therapy. If activity is measured it must be timed to assess trough or peak activity, so that results are interpreted in light of published data. Because there is more variability in peak concentrations among the DOACs, trough levels are recommended if steady-state levels are being assessed. To date, no laboratory assays developed specifically to measure DOAC activity have been approved by the Food and Drug Administration. There is no evidence to support dose adjustment based on test results.

Screening Coagulation Tests (Prothrombin Time and Activated Partial Thromboplastin Time) and Direct Oral Anticoagulants

The prothrombin time (PT) measures levels of the coagulation proteins in the classical extrinsic and common pathways (**Fig. 2**). For this assay platelet-poor plasma is prepared from sodium citrate–anticoagulated whole blood. Coagulation is activated in vitro by the addition of calcium and a thromboplastin reagent, which contains a source of tissue factor and phospholipid. The laboratory result is the time to clot formation.[13,14]

Because there is variability in sensitivity to factor deficiencies depending on the source of tissue factor and phospholipid used for the PT assay, the INR was introduced to standardize results.[13] The INR equals (patient PT/mean normal PT)[ISI]. The international sensitivity index (ISI) reflects the responsiveness of each thromboplastin

Table 1
Key drug characteristics

Drug	Drug Targets (Direct Inhibitors)	% Renal Clearance	Measured Peak Level (ng/mL)	Measured Trough Level (ng/mL)
Dabigatran	Thrombin	80[53]	175 (CV, 74%)[a]	91 (CV, 82%)[a]
Rivaroxaban	Factor Xa	36[54]	215 (22–535)[b]	32 (6–239)[b]
Apixaban	Factor Xa	25[55]	129 (CV, 10%)[c]	50 (20%)[c]
Edoxaban	Factor Xa	50[10]	n/a	36 (IQR, 19–62)[d]

Abbreviations: CV, coefficient of variation; IQR, interquartile range; n/a, not available.
[a] Mean concentration and CV in patients with atrial fibrillation on 150 mg twice daily.[9]
[b] Steady state mean in healthy volunteers given 10 mg daily with range given in parenthesis.[14]
[c] Steady state mean concentration in six healthy volunteers given 5 mg twice daily with CV given.[56]
[d] Median value in patients with atrial fibrillation given 60 mg daily with IQR given.[13]

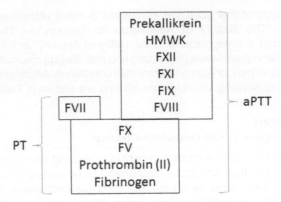

Fig. 2. Coagulation factors affecting the PT and activated partial thromboplastin time (aPTT). F, Factor; HMWK, high-molecular-weight kininogen.

reagent to reductions in the vitamin K–dependent clotting factors. Recombinant tissue factor is assigned an ISI of 1.0. It is important to remember that the ISI reflects the sensitivity to the effect of warfarin on the PT and may not reflect factor activities influenced by other drugs or medical conditions. The calculation and use of the INR using the ISI established for monitoring of warfarin anticoagulation is not valid for rivaroxaban, or other Xa inhibitors, because this has been shown to increase the drug-induced between-thromboplastin variability.[15]

The activated partial thromboplastin time (aPTT) measures levels of the coagulation proteins in the classical intrinsic and common pathways (see **Fig. 2**). The term "partial thromboplastin" was first used to describe the reagent because activation of clotting in the test did not correct the deficit in hemophilic plasma.[16] This is in contrast to the "complete thromboplastin" phospholipid and tissue factor used in the PT. In the 1960s, the addition of a surface activator (eg, silica, ellagic acid, or kaolin) became standard because it improves assay precision and sensitivity to factor deficiencies.[16] As for the PT, platelet-poor plasma prepared from sodium citrate–anticoagulated whole blood is used. Coagulation is activated in vitro by the addition of calcium and a surface activator. The laboratory result is the time to clot formation.[13,14]

DOACs differ in their effect on the PT and aPTT and neither of these assays can be used to exclude significant drug concentrations of dabigatran, rivaroxaban, or apixaban unless laboratory-specific assay sensitivity to the drug is known **(Table 2)**.[17]

Dabigatran

The aPTT and the PT have variable sensitivity to dabigatran.[18] The aPTT is more sensitive than the PT; however, there is a curvilinear dose response with a varying relationship between drug level and anticoagulant effect.[19–21] A normal aPTT or PT cannot be used to absolutely exclude an anticoagulant effect of the drug. The aPTT is usually prolonged at dabigatran concentration greater than 100 ng/mL, the approximate expected trough level in patients on therapy. The PT is typically within normal limits at a dabigatran concentration of 100 ng/mL but elevated at concentrations greater than 400 ng/mL.[20,22]

Rivaroxaban

The sensitivity of the PT to rivaroxaban varies widely by laboratory reagent used,[23–26] and for that reason a normal PT cannot be used to exclude the presence of clinically relevant anticoagulant activity unless the laboratory sensitivity of the PT reagent is

Table 2
Laboratory tests to assess and/or monitor DOAC anticoagulant activity

| Drug[a] | Clinical Scenario | | |
	Exclude Relevant Anticoagulant Effect	Detect Overanticoagulation	Monitor Drug Activity
Dabigatran	TCT	aPTT, TCT, ECA, ECT	Dilute TCT[c], ECA, ECT
Rivaroxaban	Anti-Xa[a]	PT, anti-Xa[b]	PT[d], anti-Xa[b]
Apixaban	Anti-Xa[a]	Anti-Xa[b], PT only if sensitivity established in local laboratory	Anti-Xa[b]

Abbreviations: ECA, ecarin chromogenic assay; ECT, ecarin clotting time; TCT, thrombin time.
[a] Anti-Xa assays with low-molecular-weight heparin standards can be used to exclude the presence of drug, but not to quantify drug level.
[b] Drug-specific anti-Xa.
[c] Includes HEMOCLOT assay.
[d] If calibrated in laboratory using rivaroxaban standard.

known. As examples, the reagents REcombiPlasTin (Instrumentation Laboratory, Bedford, MA) and Neoplastin (Diagnostica Stago, Parsippany, NJ) are more sensitive to rivaroxaban than Thromborel S or Innovin (both Siemens Healthcare Diagnostics, Malvern, PA).[27] The PT is prolonged with elevated drug concentrations, with the degree of elevation dependent on the sensitivity of the reagent used.

The level of rivaroxaban activity can be assessed by a PT if the test has been validated with rivaroxaban standards. Rivaroxaban plasma calibrators can be used to determine the sensitivity of the thromboplastin reagent and to standardize the assay in the individual laboratory. Rivaroxaban-specific ISI methodology is under study and seems feasible for future application.[15] Modifications of the PT (dilute PT and modified PT) to improve performance characteristics in assay of rivaroxaban-induced anticoagulation have been developed but are not widely used.

The aPTT is less sensitive to rivaroxaban than the PT and cannot be used to exclude clinically significant drug concentrations.[23–25] The aPTT is generally be prolonged in the setting of elevated rivaroxaban levels, but there is considerable variability depending on the aPTT reagent used by the laboratory.

Apixaban

The PT is less sensitive to apixaban than rivaroxaban and may be within normal limits in many patients with clinically relevant anticoagulant activity.[11,17,26–28] The PT would generally be prolonged in a patient with elevated apixaban drug concentrations, but given the low sensitivity of some PT reagents to apixaban, one cannot assume that to be true unless the sensitivity of the PT reagent to apixaban is known.[25,28] The aPTT is very insensitive to apixaban and may not be elevated, even in the setting of significantly elevated apixaban levels.[11,17,25,28]

Edoxaban

A systematic review of evidence on the effect of edoxaban on PT and aPTT was recently published.[29] Nine studies met criteria. The authors concluded that a normal PT may not exclude clinically relevant levels. The aPTT was insufficiently sensitive to edoxaban to use to measure anticoagulant activity. Morishima and Kamisato[30] documented the variable sensitivity of different PT and aPTT reagents to edoxaban.

For some thromboplastin reagents, the laboratory may be able to determine edoxaban activity using the PT when edoxaban laboratory standards become available.

Testing Direct Oral Anticoagulants Activity Using Liquid Chromatography/Tandem Mass Spectrometry Methodology

Measurement of drug activity by LC-MS/MS methodology is the gold standard for measurement of DOAC drug activity.[17] This methodology was used to measure levels in the clinical trials and it is the measurement to which other assays should be standardized. The testing is available through some commercial reference laboratories and could be used to assess steady-state levels, where laboratory results are not needed urgently.

Testing Specific for Measurement of Direct Thrombin Inhibitory Activity

Thrombin clotting time

The thrombin clotting time (TCT), or thrombin time, measures conversion of fibrinogen to fibrin by thrombin and is exquisitely sensitive to the presence of dabigatran.[20] A normal TCT can be used to exclude the presence of drug and an anticoagulant effect. In patients with therapeutic and higher range plasma concentrations, the TCT is often prolonged above the upper limit of the laboratories' testing range. A modification of the TCT, the dilute thrombin time, is used to assess the anticoagulant effect of direct thrombin inhibitors,[31] and a commercial assay, the HEMOCLOT (Hyphen BioMed), is approved for use in Europe and Canada and is used for measurement of dabigatran levels.[32]

Ecarin clotting time

An ecarin chromogenic assay or clotting time can be used to assess dabigatran activity, although these assays are not widely available. They use the venom of the saw-scaled viper *Echis carinatus* to convert prothrombin to thrombin via the intermediary meizothrombin, which is sensitive to inhibition by direct thrombin inhibitors. Ecarin clotting activity correlates directly with the dabigatran concentration.[18,33]

Direct Xa inhibitors have no effect on TCT, HEMOCLOT, or ecarin-based assays. Because dabigatran exilate is a prodrug, commercially available dabigatran-spiked plasmas are available for use in establishment of standard curves of drug concentrations. When dabigatran calibrators are used results are expressed in nanogram per milliliter of dabigatran.

Testing Specific for Measurement of Xa Inhibition

Anti-factor Xa (anti-Xa) assays

This assay is well established to measure the Xa inhibitory effect of heparins and fondaparinux.[34] To measure the inhibitory effect of these antithrombin-dependent drugs, the assay is either dependent on the antithrombin in the patient plasma or is added during the testing. Rivaroxaban, apixaban, and edoxaban do not require antithrombin for activity and thus antithrombin is not a component in the assay.

As illustrated in **Fig. 3**, for the measurement of rivaroxaban, apixaban, and edoxaban activity, factor Xa is added to the patient's plasma. The drug binds to and decreases the Xa available to react with the Xa-specific chromogenic substrate. Residual Xa activity cleaves the substrate and the color released is measured spectrophotometrically. The amount of anti-Xa activity is determined from a standard curve using drug-specific calibrators. There is an inverse relationship between the amount of Xa generated and the drug activity level.

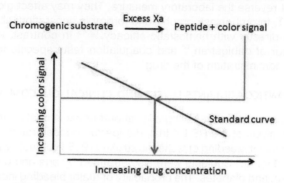

Patient plasma (with drug) + Factor Xa ⟶ Anti-Xa drug:Xa complex +Excess Xa

Chromogenic substrate $\xrightarrow{\text{Excess Xa}}$ Peptide + color signal

Fig. 3. Principle of anti-Xa assay for direct Xa inhibitor. Patient plasma containing the drug is incubated with excess factor Xa. Drug:Xa complexes are formed and excess Xa remains. Remaining Xa is assayed using a chromogenic substrate where the color generated is proportional to the Xa activity. Using a standard curve of color signal versus drug concentration, the anti-Xa drug activity is determined, as illustrated by the *arrow*.

DOAC drug-specific anti-Xa activity measurement using a drug-specific calibrator correlates well with LC-MS/MS determinations and is the assay of choice to assess rivaroxaban and apixaban levels,[26,35,36] and will be for edoxaban when a laboratory standard becomes available. Given the insensitivity of PT and aPTT to apixaban, the anti-Xa assay is key to assess apixaban activity.

Some hospital laboratories have anti-Xa assays available on a 24/7 basis, whereas in other settings it is not possible to obtain the test in an urgent manner. If the goal is to rule out the presence of rivaroxaban, apixaban, or edoxaban an anti-Xa assay using a low-molecular-weight heparin standard can be used if that is available. However, it does not quantify the amount of drug present and assays with added antithrombin overestimate the anti-Xa activity.[26,37]

Dabigatran has no effect on anti-Xa activity assays.

Other Assays for Monitoring Direct Oral Anticoagulants

Russell viper venom time

Russell viper venom activates coagulation through factor X and is used for the assessment of lupus anticoagulants.[38] The dilute Russell viper venom time, using the higher hexagonal-phase phospholipid concentration found in the dilute Russell viper venom time confirm assay, has been shown to be sensitive to dabigatran, rivaroxaban, and apixaban.[12,39] Although further study and standardization is needed, the dilute Russell viper venom time holds promise as a rapid screening assay.

Global assays

Thromboelastography and thrombin generation have been used to assess DOAC activity.[12,40,41] Although many assay parameters are affected by these drugs, they have not been standardized and the relationship between results and drug concentration is largely unknown. Further study is needed before they are used clinically to assess drug activity.

Assessing Reversal of Direct Oral Anticoagulants

Prothrombin complex concentrates and recombinant factor VIIa are sometimes used to reverse the anticoagulant effect of DOACs in patients who are bleeding or need an urgent intervention.[42] Because these products do not reverse the drug-specific activity, they do not reverse the laboratory measure. They may affect global assays, such as the PT, aPTT, thromboelastography, and thrombin generation, although results are not correlated directly with hemostatic efficacy.[12,43] In contrast, idarucizumab is a specific inhibitor of dabigatran,[44] and coagulation tests specific for dabigatran are reversed after administration of the drug.

DIRECT ORAL ANTICOAGULANTS LEVELS AND CLINICAL OUTCOMES

Limited data are available evaluating clinical outcomes in relation to drug levels. In a prespecified analysis of the RE-LY trial, dabigatran concentration was evaluated as a risk factor for major bleeding or ischemic stroke in 9183 subjects with atrial fibrillation on dabigatran (**Fig. 4**).[9] Subjects were also stratified by age and covariates included sex, prior stroke, and diabetes. The probability of major bleeding increased by decade of age and by steady state trough concentration from that study. Although the risk of recurrent stroke increased by age, there was little effect of drug concentration.

In a study of 44 patients on dabigatran, Šinigoj and colleagues[45] found that patients with bleeding had significantly higher trough drug concentrations, whereas peak concentrations had no predictive value. In analysis of patients receiving rivaroxaban in the ROCKET AF trial, major bleeding was found with increasing PT levels.[11] There was no association of PT with recurrent ischemic events. Analysis of the ENGAGE AF-TIMI 48 trial of edoxaban in atrial fibrillation demonstrated that trough levels correlated with bleeding risk.[46] Reduction in dose decreased bleeding and did not increase ischemic events.

LIMITATIONS
Influence of Direct Oral Anticoagulants on Other Coagulation Assays

Because DOACs inhibit clotting they affect many assays where the formation of a blood clot is the read out for the coagulation assay, a common end point (**Table 3**). This includes assays used to test for thrombophilia, including activity measurements antithrombin, protein C, or protein S activity, APC resistance, and lupus anticoagulant testing, and these tests should not be performed in patients on these drugs.[12,24,47–49]

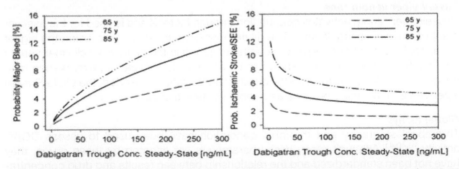

Fig. 4. Probability of clinical outcomes versus dabigatran plasma concentrations in the RE-LY trial. Major bleeding event (*left*) and ischemic stroke/systemic embolic event (SEE) (*right*) versus trough dabigatran plasma concentration in patients with atrial fibrillation by age (65, 75, and 85 years). Covariates include sex, prior stroke, and diabetes. Conc., concentration. (*From* Reilly PA, Lehr T, Haertter S, et al. The effect of dabigatran plasma concentrations and patient characteristics on the frequency of ischemic stroke and major bleeding in atrial fibrillation patients. J Am Coll Cardiol 2014;63:325; with permission.)

Table 3
Interference by DOACs in selected coagulation assays

	Dabigatran	Rivaroxaban	Apixaban
APC resistance	Increases	Increases	NR
Antithrombin	May increase[a]	May increase[b]	NR
Fibrinogen	May decrease	May increase[c]	NR
Factor activity levels	May decrease	May decrease	May decrease
Lupus anticoagulant	False positive	False positive	False positive

See text for references.
Abbreviation: NR, not reported.
[a] Overestimation with thrombin-based assays.
[b] Overestimation with FXa-based assays.
[c] Overestimation when measured by PT-derived assays; no effect in thrombin-based assays.

False-positive testing for lupus anticoagulants, even with a positive phospholipid correction step, have been reported in patients on dabigatran, rivaroxaban, and apixaban, and would be presumed to be true for edoxaban.[47–50] Chromogenic assays and measures of antigen levels or DNA-based assays should not be affected by these drugs.

Fibrinogen measurements determined by Claus methodology, the most common approach, may be artifactually lowered in the presence of dabigatran.[20,50] Fibrinogen measured using a prothrombin-based method may be artifactually elevated by all three drugs, the extent depending on the reagent used.[48] Individual clotting factor assays may also be affected.[12,51] This depends, in part, on the reagent and methodology used. Rivaroxaban has been reported to falsely lower one stage and chromogenic FVIII assays.[52] Clinicians should discuss individual assays with their laboratory to understand the potential impact of the drug on the test result.

SUMMARY

Clinicians may need to assess anticoagulant effect of DOACs. The clinical circumstance dictates the urgency for laboratory assessment and the availability of laboratory testing differs depending on the assay. The commonly available TCT can be used to exclude clinically relevant dabigatran anticoagulant activity, and if the reagent sensitivity is known, the PT can be used to exclude clinically relevant rivaroxaban concentrations. However, an anti-Xa assay is needed to exclude clinically relevant apixaban concentrations. Laboratory assay parameters for edoxaban are still being established. DOACS can affect clot-based assays, including those used to assess for thrombophilias, factor assays, and thromboelastography. Before assessing drug levels, it is important to recall that true therapeutic ranges have not been established and on-therapy drug concentrations vary widely among patients on standard therapy. Although data are accumulating correlating trough drug levels and bleeding risks, at this time there is only limited evidence to support dose adjustment based on test results.

REFERENCES

1. Connolly SJ, Ezekowitz MD, Yusuf S, et al. Dabigatran versus warfarin in patients with atrial fibrillation. N Engl J Med 2009;361:1139–51.
2. Patel MR, Mahaffey KW, Garg J, et al. Rivaroxaban versus warfarin in nonvalvular atrial fibrillation. N Engl J Med 2011;365:883–91.

3. Granger CB, Alexander JH, McMurray JJ, et al. Apixaban versus warfarin in patients with atrial fibrillation. N Engl J Med 2011;365:981–92.
4. Giugliano RP, Ruff CT, Braunwald E, et al. Edoxaban versus warfarin in patients with atrial fibrillation. N Engl J Med 2013;369:2093–104.
5. Schulman S, Kearon C, Kakkar AK, et al. Dabigatran versus warfarin in the treatment of acute venous thromboembolism. N Engl J Med 2009;361:2342–52.
6. Bauersachs R, Berkowitz SK, Brenner B, et al. Oral rivaroxaban for symptomatic venous thromboembolism. N Engl J Med 2010;363:2499–510.
7. Agnelli G, Buller HR, Cohen A, et al. Oral apixaban for the treatment of acute venous thromboembolism. N Engl J Med 2013;369:799–808.
8. Buller HR, Decousus H, Grosso MA, et al. Edoxaban versus warfarin for the treatment of symptomatic venous thromboembolism. N Engl J Med 2013;369:1406–15.
9. Reilly PA, Lehr T, Haertter S, et al. The effect of dabigatran plasma concentrations and patient characteristics on the frequency of ischemic stroke and major bleeding in atrial fibrillation patients. J Am Coll Cardiol 2014;63:321–8.
10. U.S. Food and Drug Administration. Briefing information for the September 8, 2011 meeting of the cardiovascular and renal drugs advisory committee. Available at: http://www.fda.gov/downloads/AdvisoryCommittees/CommittesMeetingMaterials/Drug/CardiovascularandRenalDRugsAdvisoryCommitttee/UCM270796.pdf. Accessed November 14, 2015.
11. Skeppholm M, Al-Aieshy F, Berndtsson M, et al. Clinical evaluation of laboratory methods to monitor apixaban treatment in patients with atrial fibrillation. Thromb Res 2015;136:148–53.
12. Favaloro EJ. Laboratory testing in the era of direct or non-vitamin K antagonist oral anticoagulants: a practical guide to measuring their activity and avoiding diagnostic errors. Semin Thromb Hemost 2015;41:208–27.
13. Bates SM, Weitz JI. Coagulation assays. Circulation 2005;112:e53–60.
14. Chandler WL. Initial evaluation of hemostasis: reagent and method selection. In: Kitchen S, Olson JD, Preston FE, editors. Quality in laboratory hemostasis and thrombosis. Hoboken (NJ): Wiley-Blackwell; 2009. p. 63–71.
15. Tripodi A, Chantarangkul V, Guinet C, et al. The international normalized ratio calibrated for rivaroxaban has the potential to normalize prothrombin time results for rivaroxaban-treated patients: results of an in vitro study. J Thromb Haemost 2011;9:226–8.
16. Owens CA. Tests of blood, plasma factors and platelets. In: Nichols WL, Bowie EJW, editors. The history of blood coagulation. Rochester (MN): Mayo Foundation for Medical Education and Research; 2001. p. 191–219.
17. Cuker A, Siegal DM, Crowther MA, et al. Laboratory measurement of the anticoagulant activity of the non-vitamin K oral anticoagulants. J Am Coll Cardiol 2014;64:1128–9.
18. Baglin T, Hillarp A, Tripodi A, et al. Measuring oral direct inhibitors of thrombin and factor Xa: a recommendation from the Subcommittee on Control of Anticoagulation of the Scientific and Standardization Committee of the International Society on Thrombosis and Haemostasis. J Thromb Haemost 2013;11:756–60.
19. van Ryn J, Stangier J, Haertter S, et al. Dabigatran etexilate: a novel, reversible, oral direct thrombin inhibitor: interpretation of coagulation assays and reversal of anticoagulant activity. Thromb Haemost 2010;103:1116–27.
20. Lindahl TL, Baghaei F, Blixter IF, et al. Effects of the oral, direct thrombin inhibitor dabigatran on five common coagulation assays. Thromb Haemost 2011;105:371–8.

21. Du S, Weiss C, Christina G, et al. Determination of dabigatran in plasma, serum, and urine samples: comparison of six methods. Clin Chem Lab Med 2015;53: 1237–47.

22. Antovic JP, Skeppholm M, Eintrei J, et al. Evaluation of coagulation assays versus LC-MS/MS for determinations of dabigatran concentrations in plasma. Eur J Clin Pharmacol 2013;69:1875–81.

23. Samama MM, Martinoli JL, LeFlem L, et al. Assessment of laboratory assays to measure rivaroxaban: an oral, direct factor Xa inhibitor. Thromb Haemost 2010; 103:815–25.

24. Hillarp A, Baghaei F, Blixter IF, et al. Effects of the oral, direct factor Xa inhibitor rivaroxaban on commonly used coagulation assays. J Thromb Haemost 2011; 9:133–9.

25. Dale BJ, Ginsberg JS, Johnston M, et al. Comparison of the effects of apixaban and rivaroxaban on prothrombin and activated partial thromboplastin times using various reagents. J Thromb Haemost 2014;12:1810–5.

26. Königsbrügge O, Quehenberger P, Belik S, et al. Anti-coagulation assessment with prothrombin time and anti-Xa assays in real-world patients on treatment with rivaroxaban. Ann Hematol 2015;94:1463–71.

27. Becker RC, Alexander JH, Newby LK, et al. Effect of apixaban, an oral and direct factor Xa inhibitor, on coagulation activity biomarkers following acute coronary syndrome. Thromb Haemost 2010;104:976–83.

28. Tripodi A, Padovan L, Testa S, et al. How the direct oral anticoagulant apixaban affects hemostatic parameters. Results of a multicenter multiplatform study. Clin Chem Lab Med 2015;53:265–73.

29. Cuker A, Husseinzadeh H. Laboratory measurement of the anticoagulant activity of edoxaban: a systemic review. J Thromb Thrombolysis 2015;39:288–94.

30. Morishima Y, Kamisato C. Laboratory measurements of the oral direct factor Xa inhibitor edoxaban: comparison of prothrombin time, activated partial thromboplastin time, thrombin generation assay. Am J Clin Pathol 2015;143:241–7.

31. Love JE, Ferrell C, Chandler WL. Monitoring direct thrombin inhibitors with a plasma diluted thrombin time. Thromb Haemost 2007;98:234–42.

32. Stangier J, Feuring M. Using the HEMOCLOT direct thrombin inhibitor assay to determine plasma concentrations of dabigatran. Blood Coagul Fibrinolysis 2012;23:138–43.

33. Nowak G. The ecarin clotting time, a universal method to quantify direct thrombin inhibitors. Pathophysiol Haemost Thromb 2004;33:173–83.

34. Hirsh J, Warkentin TE, Shaughnessy SG, et al. Heparin and low molecular weight heparin. Mechanism of action, pharmacokinetics, dosing, monitoring, efficacy and safety. Chest 2001;119:64S–94S.

35. Samama MM, Contant G, Spiro TE, et al. Evaluation of the anti-factor Xa chromogenic assay for the measurement of rivaroxaban plasma concentrations using calibrators and controls. Thromb Haemost 2012;107:379–87.

36. Harenberg J, Marx S, Weiss C, et al. Report of the subcommittee of control of anticoagulation on the determination of the anticoagulant effect of rivaroxaban. J Thromb Haemost 2012;10:1433–6.

37. Mani H, Rohde G, Stratmann G, et al. Accurate determination of rivaroxaban levels requires different calibrator sets but not addition of antithrombin. Thromb Haemost 2012;108:191–8.

38. Moore GW. Recent guidelines and recommendations for laboratory detection of lupus anticoagulants. Semin Thromb Hemost 2014;40:163–71.

39. Exner T, Ellwoood L, Rubie J, et al. Testing for new oral anticoagulants with LA-resistant Russell's viper venom reagents. An in vitro study. Thromb Haemost 2013;109:762–5.
40. Dias JD, Norem K, Doorneweerd DD. Use of thromboelastography (TEG) for detection of new oral anticoagulants. Arch Pathol Lab Med 2015;139:665–73.
41. Tripodi A, Padovan L, Chantarangkul V, et al. How the direct oral anticoagulant apixaban affects thrombin generation parameters. Thromb Res 2015;135: 1186–90.
42. Siegal DM, Garcai DA, Crowther MA. How I treat: target specific oral anticoagulant associated bleeding. Blood 2014;123:1152–8.
43. Dinkelaar J, Patiwael S, Harenberg J, et al. Global coagulation tests: their applicability for measuring direct factor Xa- and thrombin inhibition reversal of anticoagulation by prothrombin complex concentrate. Clin Chem Med 2014;52: 1615–23.
44. Pollack CV Jr, Reilly PA, Eikelboom J, et al. Idarucizumab for dabigatran reversal. N Engl J Med 2015;373:511–20.
45. Šinigoj P, Malmström RE, Vene N, et al. Dabigatran concentration: variability and potential bleeding prediction in "real-life" patients with atrial fibrillation. Basic Clin Pharmacol Toxicol 2015;117:323–9.
46. Ruff CT, Giugliano RP, Braunwald E, et al. Association between edoxaban dose, concentration, anti-factor Xa activity, and outcomes: an analysis of data from the randomized, double-blind ENGAGE AF-TIMI 48 trial. Lancet 2015;385:2288–95.
47. Funk DMA. Coagulation assays and anticoagulant monitoring. Hematology 2012; 2012:460–5.
48. Mani H. Interpretation of coagulation test results under direct oral anticoagulants. Int J Lab Hematol 2014;36:261–8.
49. Martinuzzo ME, Barrera LH, D'Adamo MA, et al. Frequent false-positive results of lupus anticoagulant tests in plasmas of patients receiving the new oral anticoagulants and enoxaparin. Int J Lab Hematol 2014;36:144–50.
50. Halbmayer WM, Weigel G, Quehenberger P, et al. Interference of the new oral anticoagulant dabigatran with frequently used coagulation tests. Clin Chem Lab Med 2013;50:1601–5.
51. Asmis LM, Alberio L, Angelillo-Scherrer A, et al. Rivaroxaban: quantification by anti-FXa assay and influence on coagulation tests. A study in 9 Swiss laboratories. Thromb Res 2012;129:492–8.
52. Tichelaar V, de Jong H, Nijland H, et al. Interference of rivaroxaban in one-stage and chromogenic factor VIII: C assays. Thromb Haemost 2011;106:990–2.
53. Stangier J, Rathgen K, Stahle H, et al. The pharmacokinetics, pharmacodynamics and tolerability of dabigatran etexilate, a new oral direct thrombin inhibitor, in male subjects. Br J Clin Pharmacol 2007;64:292–303.
54. Weinz C, Schwarz T, Kubitza D, et al. Metabolim and excretion of rivaroxaban, an oral, direct Factor Xa inhibitor, in rats, dogs and humans. Drug Metab Dispos 2009;37:1056–64.
55. Raghavean N, Frost CE, Yu Z, et al. Apixaban metabolism and pharmacokinetics after oral administration to humans. Drug Metab Dispos 2009;37:74–81.
56. Frost C, Nepal S, Wang J, et al. Safety, pharmacokinetics and pharmacodynamics of multiple oral doses of apixaban, a factor Xa inhibitor, in healthy subjects. Br J Clin Pharmacol 2013;76:776–86.

Postorthopedic Surgery Joint Replacement Surgery Venous Thromboembolism Prophylaxis

Louis M. Kwong, MD, FACS[a],*, Jon A. Kimball, MD[b]

KEYWORDS

- Thrombophrophylaxis • Rivaroxaban • Apixaban • Total hip arthroplasty
- Total knee arthroplasty • NOAC • Venous thromboembolism (VTE)

KEY POINTS

- Total hip and total knee arthroplasty put patients at high risk for venous thromboembolism.
- Significant research and development has been done in the search for the ideal postoperative thromboprophylactic agent.
- Direct factor Xa inhibitors like rivaroxaban and apixaban are novel oral anticoagulants with improved effectiveness and good safety profiles.
- Inconsistency across clinical trials with regard to the definition of trial safety endpoints has made it impossible to compare these agents with regard to bleeding.

INTRODUCTION

The performance of elective total hip arthroplasty (THA) or total knee arthroplasty (TKA) places patients at high risk for venous thromboembolism (VTE; **Tables 1 and 2**). These major orthopedic procedures contribute to all 3 components of Virchow's triad—vascular injury, stasis, and hypercoagulability. This places patients at high risk for the development of thrombosis. The subluxation of the tibia anteriorly during knee replacement surgery or the dislocation of the hip anteriorly or posteriorly in the course of hip replacement surgery imparts traction and torsional forces on blood

Disclosure Statements: ConvaTec, Iroko, Janssen, Mallinckrodt, Zimmer (consultant); Illuminoss, National Science Foundation, Stryker, Zimmer (research grant); Zimmer (royalties) (L.M. Kwong). No disclosures (J.A. Kimball).
[a] Department of Orthopaedic Surgery, Harbor-UCLA Medical Center, 1000 West Carson Street, Box 422, Torrance, CA 90509, USA; [b] Department of Orthopaedic Surgery, Harbor-UCLA Medical Center, 1000 West Carson Stree, Box 422, Torrance, CA 90509, USA
* Corresponding author.
E-mail address: lkwong@dhs.lacounty.gov

Hematol Oncol Clin N Am 30 (2016) 1007–1018
http://dx.doi.org/10.1016/j.hoc.2016.05.001
0889-8588/16/$ – see front matter © 2016 Elsevier Inc. All rights reserved.
hemonc.theclinics.com

Table 1
Incidence of VTE in hip and knee arthroplasty patients in the absence of thromboprophylaxis

Type of Surgery	Total DVT (%)	Proximal DVT (%)	Total PE (%)	Fatal PE (%)
Hip arthroplasty	42–57	18–36	0.9–28.0	0.1–2.0
Knee arthroplasty	41–85	5–22	1.5–10	0.1–1.7

Abbreviations: DVT, deep-vein thrombosis; PE, pulmonary embolism; VTE, venous thromboembolism.
    Adapted from Geerts WH, Pineo GF, Heit JA, et al. Prevention of venous thromboembolism. Chest 126;2004:351.

vessels. This can cause direct vascular endothelial damage that can initiate the process of thrombosis intraoperatively. The period of time spent immobile on the operating room table, exacerbated by use of anesthetic paralytic agents or the use of a tourniquet during knee replacement surgery, further contributes to vascular stasis. As a consequence of the patient's biologic response to tissue injury, the patient's circulatory system is showered with tissue thromboplastins, which induces a state of hypercoagulability.

As our understanding of the pathophysiology of VTE after joint arthroplasty has increased, various pharmacologic strategies have been developed to directly or indirectly target different aspects of the coagulation cascade. It has been estimated that the postoperative risk of deep vein thrombosis (DVT) without systemic anticoagulation

Table 2
Comparative efficacy of pharmacologic agents in risk reduction of deep-vein thrombosis in patients after total hip and knee arthroplasty

Pharmacologic Agent	Relative Risk Reduction (%) Compared with Placebo
Total hip arthroplasty	
Low-molecular-weight heparin	70–71
Aspirin	0–26
Warfarin	59–61
Fondaparinux[a]	45
Apixaban[b]	36
Rivaroxaban[c]	48–76
Total knee arthroplasty	
Low-molecular-weight heparin	51–52
Aspirin	0–13
Warfarin	23–27
Fondaparinux[a]	63
Apixaban[b]	38
Rivaroxaban[35]	31

[a] Odds reduction for venous thromboembolism for fondaparinux versus enoxaparinparin.[15,18,19]
[b] Cite studies for ADVANCE-1-2-3 (Apixaban Dose Orally vs ANTiCoagulation with Enoxaparin-1-2-3).
[c] Cite studies for RECORD1-3 (REgulation of Coagulation in ORthopedic surgery to prevent Deep vein thrombosis and pulmonary embolism1-3).
    Data from Geerts WH, Heit JA, Clagett GP, et al. Prevention of venous thromboembolism. Chest 2001;119(1 Suppl):132S–75S; and Gallus AS. Applying risk assessment models in orthopaedic surgery: overview of our clinical experience. Blood Coagul Fibrinolysis 1999;10(Suppl 2):S53–61.

is as high as 42% to 57% and 85% and the rates of symptomatic pulmonary embolism (PE) was as high as 0.9% to 28% and 1.5% to 10% without thromboprophylaxis after THA and TKA, respectively.[1] It has also been estimated that 45% to 80% of symptomatic VTEs occur after discharge from the hospital.[2] This stimulated significant research and development focusing on the use of in-hospital and extended duration pharmaceutical thromboprophylaxis to reduce the incidence of postoperative DVT and the possible life-threatening sequelae of PE.

According to a 2008 survey among orthopedic surgeons within the United States, there is a consensus that postoperative VTE prophylaxis should be initiated after THA or TKA.[3] However, within the United States, only 47% of THA and 61% of TKA patients are receiving postoperative VTE prophylaxis as recommended by the American College of Chest Physicians.[4] This departure from guidelines is likely multifactorial and may involve issues such as a physician's poor understanding of the American College of Chest Physicians or American Academy of Orthopaedic Surgeons guidelines as well as orthopedic surgeon concerns regarding safety.

It is acknowledged by the American Academy of Orthopaedic Surgeons and the American College of Chest Physicians that the use of routine prophylaxis for the prophylaxis against VTE is indicated in patients undergoing THA and TKA.[1,5] Dating back to the time of Sir John Charnley, the father of the modern THA, VTE was seen as an important risk to patients after hip replacement surgery.[6] Measures were taken at that time with regard to the use of systemic anticoagulation to decrease this risk. Various approaches such as unfractionated heparin and warfarin were introduced as risk reduction strategies. The use of warfarin has now been established as a standard means to reduce the risk of DVT and PE after joint arthroplasty. Although an effective strategy, the use of an established agent like warfarin has a number of disadvantages. Some patients are seemingly very warfarin sensitive, whereas others are seemingly warfarin resistant.[7–10] Also, there is no other drug used in arthroplasty surgery with as many food–drug, drug–drug, and disease–drug interactions as warfarin.[11,12] This can lead to too much or too little anticoagulation of the patient. When using warfarin, taking a careful drug inventory becomes critical to safeguard against the development of potentially serious but largely preventable complications. The requirement to dose adjust warfarin to achieve the desired international normalized ratio target also adds to the complexity of this approach and imposes an additional burden on both the patient and the surgeon. The need for phlebotomy to facilitate blood draws, laboratory analysis to determine the international normalized ratio, and a reporting requirement with associated dose adjustments are just a few of the frustrations commonly associated with warfarin. The use of warfarin after joint replacement surgery continues within the United States, but is used infrequently in other countries.[4]

Low-molecular-weight heparins (LMWHs) were investigated in the 1980s to address some of the deficiencies and disadvantages associated with the use of warfarin. LMWHs offered more predictable pharmacokinetics and pharmacodynamics.[13,14] LMWHs of all types (eg, enoxaparin, dalteparen) have been used with great success. They have proven to have good efficacy, a good safety profile, and have eliminated the need for hematologic monitoring. As an alternative to LMWHs, fondaparinux (Arixtra, GlaxoSmithKline) was developed as an indirect inhibitor of factor Xa.[15] This drug represented the pentasaccharide sequence of heparin. It acts on antithrombin, resulting in a conformational change, leading to irreversible binding to factor Xa. With a long half-life of approximately 17 hours in patients with normal renal function, fondaparinux is a true once a day dosing agent.[16–19] However, concerns regarding its safety in terms of major bleeding in the TKA trials, and the continued need for an injectable route of administration hampered the more widespread use of fondaparinux.[20] The injectable route of administration required for this drug as well as for LMWHs also highlighted the issue of patient noncompliance without appropriate patient instruction.[21] This may be in part owing to this noxious route of administration as compared with an oral route of administration.

Although a number of pharmacologic agents have been found to be effective in decreasing the risk of VTE, each agent has proven to have varying risk/benefit profiles for both the patient and the physician. The ideal thromboprophylactic agent would have the properties of an oral route of administration, a rapid onset of action, a wide therapeutic window, little or no variability in dose response, little or no interactions with food or other drugs, a predictable pharmacokinetic/pharmacodynamics profiles, no routine coagulation monitoring, no required dose adjustments, effective in reducing the risk of thromboembolic events, and a good safety profile in terms of renal, hepatic, cardiac, and hematologic complications such as bleeding.[22]

In 2011 and 2014, the US Food and Drug Administration approved rivaroxaban (Xarelto, Bayer) and apixaban (Eliquis, Bristol-Meyers Squibb), respectively, as new oral antithrombotic agents in the class of drugs known as "direct factor Xa inhibitors," to reduce the risk of DVT and PE after hip and knee replacement surgery. These agents, also known as novel oral anticoagulants (NOACs), have become increasingly popular owing to their ease of administration, effectiveness in reducing the risk of postoperative DVT and PE, a relatively low incidence of postoperative bleeding and/or wound complications, and the lack of the need for hematologic monitoring to ensure therapeutic dosing. These qualities make rivaroxaban and apixaban ideal choices for decreasing the risk of VTE after hip and knee replacement surgery.

HISTORY OF FACTOR XA INHIBITORS

Factor Xa is well-known for its enzymatic conversion of prothrombin to thrombin in the coagulation cascade. The importance of factor Xa was recognized when studying individuals with factor X deficiency.[23–25] However, it was not until two naturally occurring factor Xa inhibitors, Antistasis and Tick Anticoagulant Peptide, were isolated from the Mexican leech[26,27] and the soft tick,[28] respectively, that the potential of factor Xa inhibitors became a reality. The discovery of these naturally occurring compounds stimulated research directed toward the development of direct inhibitors of factor Xa. The investigational drugs DX-9065a[29,30] and YM-60828[31] were two of the first synthetic factor Xa inhibitors to be studied. However, these drugs demonstrated poor bioavailability and were overshadowed eventually by the concurrent research on unfractionated heparin and LMWHs. Although LMWHs had set a new standard for DVT prophylaxis, there were still several aspects of these agents such as poor bioavailability and requirement for subcutaneous administration—adversely impacting patient compliance—that left room for further research and development of the "ideal" agent for the prophylaxis against VTE. This led to the birth of several other factor Xa inhibitors including rivaroxaban and apixaban.

Rivaroxaban (Xarelto), systematic (IUPAC) name (S)-5-chloro-N-{[2-oxo-3-[4-(3-oxomorpholin-4-yl) phenyl]oxazolidin-5-yl]methyl} thiophene-2-carboxamide, developed by Bayer, was approved by the European Union in 2008 and by the United States in 2011 for use as an oral direct inhibitor of factor Xa for the prevention of DVT that may lead to PE after THA and TKA. The approval of this agent was the result of the RECORD (REgulation of Coagulation in ORthopedic surgery to prevent DVT and PE) clinical trials, which were carried out from 2008 to 2009.[32–36] These large randomized, double-blind, prospective studies were conducted to compare the efficacy and safety of rivaroxaban against the active comparator—enoxaparin—after total hip or knee replacement surgery (**Fig. 1**).

Brief Summary of REgulation of Coagulation in ORthopedic Surgery to Prevent Deep Vein Thrombosis and Pulmonary Embolism Trials

REgulation of Coagulation in ORthopedic surgery to prevent Deep vein thrombosis and pulmonary embolism 1

This phase III multicenter trial enrolled 4541 individuals to compare the efficacy and safety of rivaroxaban 10 mg every day for 35 days against the European regimen of enoxaparin 40 mg begun with a preoperative dose administered 12 hours before surgery and continued postoperatively every day for 35 days for the prevention of VTE after THA. The primary efficacy outcome (a composite of nonfatal PE, any DVT, and all-cause mortality) occurred in 1.1% and 3.7% in the rivaroxaban and enoxaparin groups, respectively (*P*<.001), representing a 71% relative risk reduction (RRR) with rivaroxaban as compared with enoxaparin. With regard to the secondary efficacy outcome of major VTE (symptomatic VTE and VTE-related death), there was a 91% RRR with the use of rivaroxaban compared with enoxaparin. There was no difference in the rate of symptomatic VTE alone. This study demonstrated similar bleeding risk profiles between the two agents.

REgulation of Coagulation in ORthopedic surgery to prevent Deep vein thrombosis and pulmonary embolism 2

This phase III multicenter trial enrolled 2509 individuals to compare the efficacy and safety of extended thromboprophylaxis with rivaroxaban 10 mg by mouth every day for 31 to 39 days to the more commonly used shorter term European regimen of enoxaparin 40 mg subcutaneously every day for 10 to 14 days after THA. The primary efficacy outcome (nonfatal PE, any DVT, and all-cause mortality) occurred in 2.0% and 8.4% in the rivaroxaban and enoxaparin groups, respectively (*P*<.001), representing a 76% RRR with the use of rivaroxaban compared with enoxaparin, demonstrating superior efficacy of extended duration thromboprophylaxis with rivaroxaban compared with shorter duration enoxaparin. With regard to major VTE, there was an 87% RRR with the use of rivaroxaban. The rate of symptomatic VTE was 0.3% and 1.3% for rivaroxaban and enoxaparin, respectively (*P*<.0040). This study also suggested similar bleeding risk profiles between the two agents.

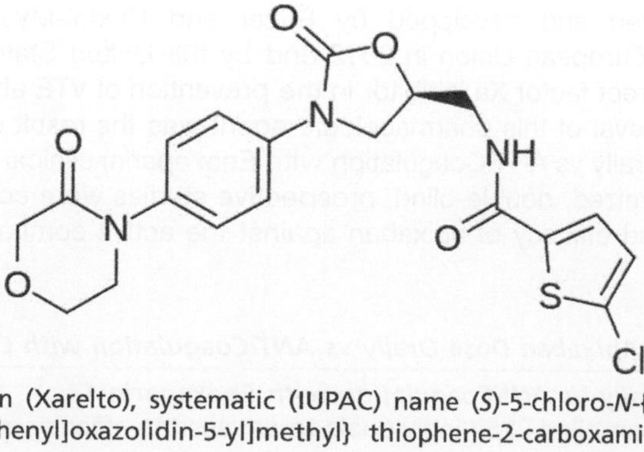

Fig. 1. Rivaroxaban (Xarelto), systematic (IUPAC) name (*S*)-5-chloro-*N*-{[2-oxo-3-[4-(3-oxo-morpholin-4-yl) phenyl]oxazolidin-5-yl]methyl} thiophene-2-carboxamide, developed by Bayer.

REgulation of Coagulation in ORthopedic surgery to prevent Deep vein thrombosis and pulmonary embolism 3

This multicenter phase III trial enrolled 2531 individuals to compare the efficacy and safety of rivaroxaban 10 mg every day for 10 to 14 days to enoxaparin 40 mg every day subcutaneously for 10 to 14 days. The primary efficacy outcome (nonfatal PE, any DVT, and all-cause mortality) occurred in 9.6% and 18.9% in the rivaroxaban and enoxaparin groups, respectively ($P<.001$), representing a 48% RRR with the use of rivaroxaban compared with enoxaparin. With regard to major VTE, there was a 60% RRR with the use of rivaroxaban. The rate of symptomatic VTE was 0.7% and 2.0% for rivaroxaban and enoxaparin respectively ($P = .005$). This study suggested similar bleeding risk profiles between the two agents.

REgulation of Coagulation in ORthopedic surgery to prevent Deep vein thrombosis and pulmonary embolism 4

This multicenter phase III trial enrolled 3148 individuals to compare the efficacy and safety of rivaroxaban 10 mg every day for 10 to 14 days against the North American regimen of enoxaparin 30 mg every 12 hours subcutaneously initiated 12 to 24 hours postoperatively for 10 to 14 days. The primary efficacy outcome (nonfatal PE, any DVT, and all-cause mortality) occurred in 6.9% and 10.1% in the rivaroxaban and enoxaparin groups, respectively ($P<.0118$), representing a RRR of 31% with the use of rivaroxaban. The rate of symptomatic VTE was 0.7% and 1.2% for rivaroxaban and enoxaparin, respectively ($P = .1868$). This study suggested similar bleeding risk profiles between the two agents, as well as superiority in reducing major VTE. This is the first clinical trial to demonstrate superiority of any antithrombotic in reducing the risk of VTE against the North American regimen of enoxaparin.

A pooled analysis of the 4 RECORD trials demonstrated superiority of rivaroxaban in reducing the incidence of the composite of symptomatic VTE and all-cause mortality after THA or TKA when compared with the study regimens of enoxaparin (0.5% vs 1.0%, respectively) in the day 12 $\pm$ 2 total active treatment period pool. This represented an RRR of 52% with the use of rivaroxaban. In the total treatment duration pool (the planned treatment period for the double-blind administration of study medication for each RECORD study), there was also a significant reduction of the composite of symptomatic VTE and all-cause mortality with the use of rivaroxaban compared with enoxaparin (0.6% vs 1.3%) and represented an RRR of 58%. The pooled analysis also demonstrated a significant reduction in the incidence of symptomatic VTE in the total treatment duration pool.[36]

Apixiban (Eliquis), systematic (IUPAC) name 1-(4-methoxyphenyl)-7-oxo-6-[4-(2-oxopiperidin-1-yl)phenyl]-4,5,6,7-tetrahydro-1*H*-pyrazolo[3,4-c]pyridine-3-carboxamide, manufactured and developed by Pfizer and Bristol-Myers Squibb, was approved by the European Union in 2012 and by the United States in 2014 to be used as an oral direct factor Xa inhibitor in the prevention of VTE after TKA and THA surgery. The approval of this pharmacologic agent was the result of the ADVANCE (Apixaban Dose Orally vs ANTiCoagulation with Enoxaparin) clinical trials.[37–39] These multicenter randomized, double-blind, prospective studies were conducted to evaluate the safety and efficacy of apixaban against the active comparator enoxaparin (**Fig. 2**).

Brief Summary of Apixaban Dose Orally vs ANTiCoagulation with Enoxaparin Trials

Apixaban Dose orally Vs ANTiCoagulation with Enoxaparin-1

This phase III trial enrolled 2287 individuals to assess the efficacy and safety of apixaban 2.5 mg by mouth twice daily starting 12 to 24 hours after surgery for 10 to 14 days

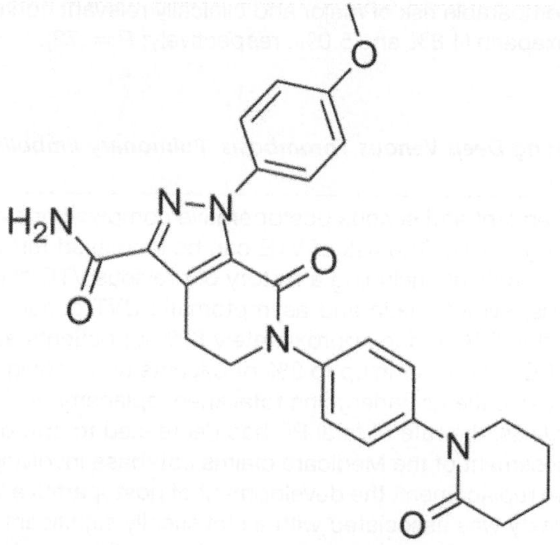

Fig. 2. Apixiban (Eliquis), systematic (IUPAC) name 1-(4-methoxyphenyl)-7-oxo-6-[4-(2-oxo-piperidin-1-yl)phenyl]-4,5,6,7-tetrahydro-1H-pyrazolo[3,4-c]pyridine-3-carboxamide, manu-factured and developed by Pfizer and Bristol-Myers Squibb.

compared with enoxaparin 30 mg subcutaneously every 12 hours starting 12 to 24 hours after surgery for 10 to 14 days after total knee replacement surgery. The primary efficacy outcome (the composite of all VTE and death owing to any cause) was 9.0% and 8.8% in the apixaban and enoxaparin groups, respectively (P = .06), and failed to meet the threshold for noninferiority of apixaban against enoxaparin. This study demonstrated a 2.9% and 4.3% (P = .03) risk of major and clinically relevant bleeds for apixaban and enoxaparin, respectively. Apixaban was found to be superior to enoxaparin for major and clinically relevant nonmajor bleeding episodes.

Apixaban Dose orally Vs ANtiCoagulation with Enoxaparin-2
This phase III trial enrolled 1973 individuals to assess the efficacy and safety of apixaban 2.5 mg by mouth twice daily starting 12 to 24 hours after surgery for 10 to 14 days compared with enoxaparin 40 mg subcutaneously once daily starting 12 hours before surgery for 10 to 14 days after TKA. The primary efficacy outcome (symptomatic and asymptomatic DVT, nonfatal PE, and all-cause death) was 15.1% and 24.4% in the apixaban and enoxaparin groups, respectively (P<.001), demonstrating the superiority of apixaban, with a RRR of 38%. This study also demonstrated a 3.5% and 4.8% (P = .0881) risk of major and clinically relevant bleeds for apixaban and enoxaparin, respectively. Major or clinically relevant nonmajor bleeding occurred in 53 of 1501 patients (4%) receiving apixaban and 72 of 1508 (5%) treated with enoxaparin (P = .09). Apixaban was found to offer a convenient and more effective alternative to enoxaparin without a significant increase in bleeding risk.

Apixaban Dose orally Vs ANtiCoagulation with Enoxaparin-3
This phase III clinical trial enrolled 1949 individuals to assess the efficacy and safety of apixaban 2.5 mg by mouth twice daily starting 12 to 24 hours after surgery for 35 days compared with enoxaparin 40 mg subcutaneously every 12 hours starting 12 hours before surgery for 35 days after THA. The primary outcome (any VTE and all-cause death) was 1.4% and 3.9% in the apixaban and enoxaparin groups, respectively (P<.001), demonstrating noninferiority and superiority of apixaban and a RRR of 36%. This study

demonstrated a comparable risk of major and clinically relevant nonmajor bleeding for apixaban and enoxaparin (4.8% and 5.0%, respectively; $P = .72$).

DISCUSSION
Efficacy in Preventing Deep Venous Thrombosis, Pulmonary Embolism, and/or All-Cause Mortality

One of the most frequent and serious postoperative complications after elective joint replacement surgery is VTE. The risk of VTE can be increased further by associated comorbidities of the patient, including a history of previous VTE.[40] In the absence of thromboprophylaxis, symptomatic and asymptomatic DVT occurs in approximately 50% of patients after THA and in approximately 60% of patients after TKA. Without prophylaxis, fatal PE may occur in up to 2% of patients undergoing total hip replacement in up to 1.7% of patients undergoing total knee replacement.[41] Since the advent of thromboprophylaxis, the rate of fatal PE has decreased to approximately 0.1% to 0.2%.[41] In an assessment of the Medicare claims database involving patients undergoing hip and knee replacement, the development of postoperative VTE after total hip and knee arthroplasty was associated with a statistically significant increase in complications including mortality, postoperative bleeding, and the need for rehospitalization within 30 days of surgery.[42]

There are an estimated 7 million individuals currently ambulating within the United States with a THA or TKA. It has been estimated that there will be a 174% and 673% increase in demand for THA and TKA, respectively, by 2030.[43,44] With such a high prevalence of joint replacement surgery, even low rates of DVT, PE, and all-cause postoperative mortality represent a significant morbidity and mortality burden on the American population. For this reason, VTE, PE, and death are important primary endpoints for any clinical trial leading to approval by the US Food and Drug Administration.

Safety

The definition of safety in terms of major bleeding, minor bleeding, and clinically relevant nonmajor bleeding has varied significantly from trial to trial with no universally accepted standard definitions. As a result, it is difficult, if not impossible, to draw any conclusions from side-to-side drug comparisons by attempting to compare safety data among various reported trials in the peer-reviewed literature.[45,46] That being said, postoperative bleeding complications seem to be of greatest concern to orthopedic surgeons.[3,47] Postoperative bleeding can lead to hemarthrosis and resultant arthrofibrosis, compromised wound healing, and increase the risk of postoperative infection and/or wound dehiscence. Surgeon concerns regarding bleeding may be adversely impacting the decision making of some physicians regarding the use of thromboprophylaxis. Data on an association between surgical site bleeding and subsequent postoperative joint or wound infection along with risk factors for bleeding (except for investigational new drug safety reports from drug vs drug clinical trials) are limited. Scarce evidence exists to implicate surgical site bleeding as a mediating factor in any hypothesized association between thromboprophylaxis and postoperative prosthetic joint infection. The validity of any such assertion is weakened by inconsistencies in reported findings and the methodologic limitations of published studies. A published review of the literature demonstrates conflicting reports with no clear association between bleeding, infection, and thromboprophylaxis.[48] Studies designed to examine specifically the causality of the interrelationship between anticoagulation prophylaxis, increased surgical site bleeding, and the risk for postoperative joint infection after total hip and knee arthroplasty are needed. Careful evaluation of pivotal clinical trials also confirms the variable definitions for postoperative bleeding. Attempts have been made to standardize the definition of bleeding so that trial to trial comparisons can more easily be made.[46] However, these recommendations have not yet been adopted.

Based on a survey conducted among members of the arthroplasty community, surgeon concerns with regard to bleeding have led to non–evidence-based approaches to VTE thromboprophylaxis by some practioners.[3] Some of the non–evidenced-based practices used include using otherwise effective agents in an unproven or ineffective manner (eg, very low dose unmonitored warfarin), or the use of agents of unproven efficacy (eg, aspirin 81 mg every day). Some have advocated that it is the timing of the first dose of antithrombotic agent that plays a more important role in the development of postoperative bleeding complications than the properties of the drug itself. The use of postoperative thromboprophylaxis is a balance between efficacy and safety. The closer the administration of the first dose of agent to the time of surgery is associated with increasing efficacy, but with the consequence of a degradation in safety with regard to bleeding complications. A delay in administration of the first dose is associated with improvements in safety from a bleeding standpoint, but is also associated with a deterioration in efficacy as reflected by an increase in venous thromboembolic events.[49] The use of NOACs is not immune to the effects of too early or too late administration of the antithrombotic agent. A guiding principle in the timing of administration of the first dose of drug is not to reference the initiation of the agent with regard to the end of surgery, but with regard to the time at which primary hemostasis has been achieved. In a very straightforward, uncomplicated, primary total joint arthroplasty, the time of primary hemostasis may correspond to the time of wound closure. However, for more complex surgeries, the time at which primary hemostasis is achieved may be many hours postoperatively. In more complicated arthroplasty surgeries, such as revision arthroplasty cases or primary joint replacements in patients with severe deformities, or in large patients who are very muscular or obese, the surgical trauma induced is more extensive. In these patients, wound channels are larger, the surgical dissection is more extensive, there are a greater number of soft tissue releases, and the instrumenting of the bone is more extensive—all leading to an increased risk of both intraoperative as well as postoperative bleeding. Because these patients will typically have closed surgical suction drains placed into the wound for the evacuation of what would otherwise accumulate as hematoma, the achievement of primary hemostasis is determined by postoperative drain output. The responsibility, therefore, falls on the operating surgeon to determine and to explicitly specify the timing of the initiation of the first dose of any antithrombotic agent based on their judgment as to the achievement of postoperative primary wound hemostasis. With regard to the NOACs, this would be 6 to 10 hours after the achievement of primary wound hemostasis for rivaroxaban, and 12 to 24 hours after the achievement of primary wound hemostasis for apixaban.

Overall, as a class of antithrombotic agents, the NOACs offer a convenient oral route of administration, proven efficacy in reducing the risk of VTE, and a good safety profile comparable to enoxaparin. With both agents used at a fixed dose without the need for monitoring, the simplified regimens increase the ease of use of postoperative thromboprophylaxis for both the patient as well as the surgeon.

REFERENCES

1. Geerts WH, Bergqvist D, Pineo GF, et al. Prevention of venous thromboembolism: American College of Chest Physicians evidence-based clinical practice guidelines (8th edition). Chest 2008;133:381S–453S.

2. Muntz J. Thromboprophylaxis in orthopedic surgery: how long is long enough? Am J Orthop (Belle Mead NJ) 2009;38:394–401.
3. Anderson FA, Huang W, Friedman RJ, et al. Prevention of venous thromboembolism after hip or knee arthroplasty: findings from a 2008 survey of US orthopedic surgeons. J Arthroplasty 2012;27:659–66.e5.
4. Friedman RJ, Gallus AS, Cushner FD, et al. Physician compliance with guidelines for deep-vein thrombosis prevention in total hip and knee arthroplasty. Curr Med Res Opin 2008;24:87–97.
5. OrthoGuidelines [WWW Document], n.d. Available at: http://www.orthoguidelines.org/topic?id=1006. Accessed February 1, 2016.
6. Crawford WJ, Hillman F, Charnley J. A clinical trial of prophylactic anticoagulant therapy in elective hip surgery. Internal Publication No. 14, Centre for Hip Surgery, Wrightington Hospital. 1968.
7. Kazi DS, Hlatky MA. Warfarin, genes, and the (health care) environment. JAMA Intern Med 2014;174:1338–9.
8. Self TH, Wallace JL, Sakaan S, et al. Effect of body weight on dose of vitamin K antagonists. South Med J 2015;108:637–43.
9. Stergiopoulos K, Brown DL. Genotype-guided vs clinical dosing of warfarin and its analogues: meta-analysis of randomized clinical trials. JAMA Intern Med 2014;174:1330–8.
10. Verhoef TI, Redekop WK, Daly AK, et al. Pharmacogenetic-guided dosing of coumarin anticoagulants: algorithms for warfarin, acenocoumarol and phenprocoumon. Br J Clin Pharmacol 2014;77:626–41.
11. Holbrook AM, Pereira JA, Labiris R, et al. Systematic overview of warfarin and its drug and food interactions. Arch Intern Med 2005;165:1095–106.
12. Zhang K, Young C, Berger J. Administrative claims analysis of the relationship between warfarin use and risk of hemorrhage including drug-drug and drug-disease interactions. J Manag Care Pharm 2006;12:640–8.
13. Bara L, Samama M. Pharmacokinetics of low molecular weight heparins. Acta Chir Scand Suppl 1988;543:65–72.
14. Verstraete M. Pharmacotherapeutic aspects of unfractionated and low molecular weight heparins. Drugs 1990;40:498–530.
15. Turpie AG, Bauer KA, Eriksson BI, et al. Fondaparinux vs enoxaparin for the prevention of venous thromboembolism in major orthopedic surgery: a meta-analysis of 4 randomized double-blind studies. Arch Intern Med 2002;162:1833–40.
16. Reynolds NA, Perry CM, Scott LJ. Fondaparinux sodium: a review of its use in the prevention of venous thromboembolism following major orthopaedic surgery. Drugs 2004;64:1575–96.
17. Turpie AG, Gallus AS, Hoek JA, et al. A synthetic pentasaccharide for the prevention of deep-vein thrombosis after total hip replacement. N Engl J Med 2001;344:619–25.
18. Turpie AG, Bauer KA, Eriksson BI, et al, PENTATHALON 2000 Study Steering Committee. Postoperative fondaparinux versus postoperative enoxaparin for prevention of venous thromboembolism after elective hip-replacement surgery: a randomised double-blind trial. Lancet 2002;359:1721–6.
19. Turpie AG, Eriksson BI, Lassen MR, et al. A meta-analysis of fondaparinux versus enoxaparin in the prevention of venous thromboembolism after major orthopaedic surgery. J South Orthop Assoc 2002;11:182–8.
20. Patel VP, Walsh M, Sehgal B, et al. Factors associated with prolonged wound drainage after primary total hip and knee arthroplasty. J Bone Joint Surg Am 2007;89:33–8.

21. Colwell CW, Pulido P, Hardwick ME, et al. Patient compliance with outpatient prophylaxis: an observational study. Orthopedics 2005;28:143–7.
22. Perzborn E, Roehrig S, Straub A, et al. The discovery and development of rivaroxaban, an oral, direct factor Xa inhibitor. Nat Rev Drug Discov 2011;10:61–75.
23. Brown DL, Kouides PA. Diagnosis and treatment of inherited factor X deficiency. Haemophilia 2008;14:1176–82.
24. Hougie C, Barrow EM, Graham JB. Stuart clotting defect. I. Segregation of an hereditary hemorrhagic state from the heterogeneous group heretofore called stable factor (SPCA, proconvertin, factor VII) deficiency. J Clin Invest 1957;36:485–96.
25. Telfer TP, Denson KW, Wright DR. A new coagulation defect. Br J Haematol 1956;2:308–16.
26. Nutt E, Gasic T, Rodkey J, et al. The amino acid sequence of antistasin. A potent inhibitor of factor Xa reveals a repeated internal structure. J Biol Chem 1988;263:10162–7.
27. Tuszynski GP, Gasic TB, Gasic GJ. Isolation and characterization of antistasin. An inhibitor of metastasis and coagulation. J Biol Chem 1987;262:9718–23.
28. Waxman L, Smith DE, Arcuri KE, et al. Tick anticoagulant peptide (TAP) is a novel inhibitor of blood coagulation factor Xa. Science 1990;248:593–6.
29. Becker RC, Alexander J, Dyke CK, et al. Development of DX-9065a, a novel direct factor Xa antagonist, in cardiovascular disease. Thromb Haemost 2004;92:1182–93.
30. Taniuchi Y, Sakai Y, Hisamichi N, et al. Biochemical and pharmacological characterization of YM-60828, a newly synthesized and orally active inhibitor of human factor Xa. Thromb Haemost 1998;79:543–8.
31. Sato K, Kawasaki T, Taniuchi Y, et al. YM-60828, a novel factor Xa inhibitor: separation of its antithrombotic effects from its prolongation of bleeding time. Eur J Pharmacol 1997;339:141–6.
32. Eriksson BI, Borris LC, Friedman RJ, et al, RECORD1 Study Group. Rivaroxaban versus enoxaparin for thromboprophylaxis after hip arthroplasty. N Engl J Med 2008;358:2765–75.
33. Kakkar AK, Brenner B, Dahl OE, et al. Extended duration rivaroxaban versus short-term enoxaparin for the prevention of venous thromboembolism after total hip arthroplasty: a double-blind, randomised controlled trial. Lancet 2008;372:31–9.
34. Lassen MR, Ageno W, Borris LC, et al. Rivaroxaban versus enoxaparin for thromboprophylaxis after total knee arthroplasty. N Engl J Med 2008;358:2776–86.
35. Turpie AG, Lassen MR, Davidson BL, et al. Rivaroxaban versus enoxaparin for thromboprophylaxis after total knee arthroplasty (RECORD4): a randomised trial. Lancet 2009;373:1673–80.
36. Turpie AG, Lassen MR, Eriksson BI, et al. Rivaroxaban for the prevention of venous thromboembolism after hip or knee arthroplasty. Pooled analysis of four studies. Thromb Haemost 2011;105:444–53.
37. Lassen MR, Gallus A, Raskob GE, et al. Apixaban versus enoxaparin for thromboprophylaxis after hip replacement. N Engl J Med 2010;363:2487–98.
38. Lassen MR, Raskob GE, Gallus A, et al. Apixaban versus enoxaparin for thromboprophylaxis after knee replacement (ADVANCE-2): a randomised double-blind trial. Lancet 2010;375:807–15.
39. Lassen MR, Raskob GE, Gallus A, et al. Apixaban or enoxaparin for thromboprophylaxis after knee replacement. N Engl J Med 2009;361:594–604.

40. Agnelli G. Prevention of venous thromboembolism in surgical patients. Circulation 2004;110:IV4–12.
41. Geerts WH, Pineo GF, Heit JA, et al. Prevention of venous thromboembolism: the Seventh ACCP Conference on Antithrombotic and Thrombolytic Therapy. Chest 2004;126:338S–400S.
42. Baser O, Supina D, Sengupta N, et al. Impact of postoperative venous thromboembolism on Medicare recipients undergoing total hip replacement or total knee replacement surgery. Am J Health Syst Pharm 2010;67:1438–45.
43. Kurtz S, Ong K, Lau E, et al. Projections of primary and revision hip and knee arthroplasty in the United States from 2005 to 2030. J Bone Joint Surg Am 2007;89: 780–5.
44. Maradit Kremers H, Larson DR, Crowson CS, et al. Prevalence of total hip and knee replacement in the United States. J Bone Joint Surg Am 2015;97:1386–97.
45. Dahl OE, Huisman MV. Dabigatran etexilate: advances in anticoagulation therapy. Expert Rev Cardiovasc Ther 2010;8(6):771–4.
46. Schulman S, Angerås U, Bergqvist D, et al. Definition of major bleeding in clinical investigations of antihemostatic medicinal products in surgical patients. J Thromb Haemost 2010;8:202–4.
47. Colwell CW Jr. Thrombosis prevention in lower extremity arthroplasty: mobile compression device or pharmacological therapy. Surg Technol Int 2014;25: 233–8.
48. Kwong LM, Kistler KD, Mills R, et al. Thromboprophylaxis, bleeding and postoperative prosthetic joint infection in total hip and knee arthroplasty: a comprehensive literature review. Expert Opin Pharmacother 2012;13:333–44.
49. Falck-Ytter Y, Francis CW, Johanson NA, et al. Prevention of VTE in orthopedic surgery patients: antithrombotic therapy and prevention of thrombosis, 9th ed: American College of Chest Physicians Evidence-Based Clinical Practice Guidelines. Chest 2012;141:e278S–325S.

Non-Vitamin K Antagonist Oral Anticoagulants in Atrial Fibrillation

 CrossMark

Anna Plitt, MD[a], Christian T. Ruff, MD, MPH[b],
Robert P. Giugliano, MD, SM[b],*

KEYWORDS

- Atrial fibrillation • NOAC • Dabigatran • Rivaroxaban • Apixaban • Edoxaban

KEY POINTS

- Non–vitamin K antagonist oral anticoagulants (NOACs) are effective in preventing stroke and systemic embolic events in patients with atrial fibrillation and have a superior safety profile compared to warfarin.
- Analyses in special populations allow for a versatile use of NOACs.
- Reversal agents for Factor Xa inhibitors are in the final stages of development; a reversal agent for dabigatran is now available.

INTRODUCTION
Atrial Fibrillation: Definition and Epidemiology

Atrial fibrillation (AF) is the most common cardiac arrhythmia with an incidence of 28 per 1000 person-years in the United States.[1] It is estimated that by 2050, the number of patients with AF will increase by 2.5 fold, affecting 6 to 12 million Americans.[2]

The causes of AF are multifactorial, and it is a challenging disease to manage. It is associated with 5-fold increased risk of stroke, 3-fold increased risk of heart failure, and 2-fold increased risk of dementia and mortality.[3] AF is also associated with multiple readmissions and hospitalizations as well as more than 99,000 deaths with an

Disclosures: A. Plitt reports no conflict of interest. Dr R.P. Giugliano reports receiving consulting fees from the American College of Cardiology, Boehringer-Ingelheim, Bristol-Myers Squibb, Daiichi Sankyo, Janssen Pharmaceuticals, Merck, Portola, and Pfizer; lecture fees from Bristol-Myers Squibb, Daiichi Sankyo, Merck, and Sanofi; and grant support through his institution from Daiichi Sankyo and Merck. Dr C.T. Ruff reports receiving consulting fees from Bayer, Daiichi Sankyo, Portola, and Boehringer Ingelheim and grant support through his institution from Daiichi Sankyo, Astra Zeneca, Eisai, and Intarcia.
a Department of Internal Medicine, Mount Sinai Hospital, One Gustave L. Levy Place, New York, NY 10029-6574, USA; b Cardiovascular Division, TIMI Study Group, Brigham and Women's Hospital, 350 Longwood Avenue, 1st Floor Offices, Boston, MA 02115, USA
* Corresponding author.
E-mail address: rgiugliano@partners.org

Hematol Oncol Clin N Am 30 (2016) 1019–1034
http://dx.doi.org/10.1016/j.hoc.2016.05.002
0889-8588/16/$ – see front matter © 2016 Elsevier Inc. All rights reserved.

hemonc.theclinics.com

estimated national incremental cost of $26 billion annually for a patient with AF versus no AF.[3,4]

Based on the findings from the Central Registry of the German Competence NETwork on Atrial Fibrillation (AFNET) study, the most common symptoms in patients with AF include chest pain, palpitations, dyspnea, dizziness, and fatigue.[5] AF can also lead to tachycardia-induced cardiomyopathy.[6] Although AF remains a significant risk factor for stroke, other underlying causes of stroke, such as local plaque rupture, atherothrombotic emboli from intracranial and extracranial arteries, carotid dissection, and presence of inflammation and coagulopathies, should be considered. This article focuses on stroke prevention using oral anticoagulants in AF.

AF is classified based on the duration of episodes.[3] The pivotal trials that compared Non-Vitamin K antagonist oral anticoagulants (NOACs) with warfarin enrolled patients with nonvalvular AF (NVAF). However, the definition of NVAF has varied between the trials; there is a lack of consensus on the definition of *valvular* and *nonvalvular* among various guidelines. Nonetheless, it is well established that the risk of thromboembolism is particularly high in AF associated with moderate to severe mitral stenosis and mechanical valves. Furthermore, it remains unknown whether the pathogenesis of thrombogenesis is different in these conditions versus other forms of AF; thus, it has been proposed to keep "mechanical and rheumatic mitral valvular AF" separate from other types of AF.[7]

AF occurs when there is a change in the atrial architecture promoting propagation and maintenance of abnormal electrical activity (**Fig. 1**). Conditions such as hypertension, coronary artery disease, and various cardiomyopathies on a cellular level are characterized by fibrosis, inflammation, and hypertrophy, which predispose to AF.[3] AF itself leads to further changes in the left atrium, endothelial damage, myocytic hypertrophy, necrosis, and mononuclear cell infiltrates, all of which predispose a patient to a hypercoagulable state.[8] Multiple genes have also been identified that predispose to AF. Most of the mutations in AF are gain-of-function mutations in potassium channels that lead to increased probability of channel opening, which in turn increase atrial action potential duration and atrial refractory period. Loss-of-function mutations in potassium channels lead to early after-depolarizations and AF.[9] Currently genome-wide

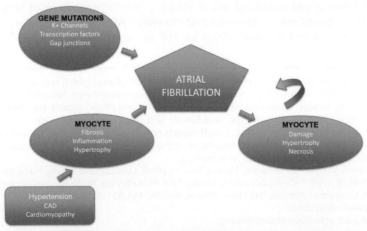

Fig. 1. Risk factors and pathophysiology of atrial fibrillation (AF). Multiple genetic, cellular, and extracardiac risk factors contribute to development of AF. CAD, coronary artery disease; K+, potassium ion.

association studies have identified numerous genes that encode gap junctions, transcription factors involved in sodium homeostasis, and cardiac transcription factors that play a role in AF.[10] It is hypothesized that ectopic atrial foci composed of atrial myocardial fibers around pulmonary veins are particularly arrhythmogenic. Pulmonary vein myocytes have been shown to reduce upstroke velocity and decrease resting membrane potential associated with delayed rectified current and decreased action potential duration.[11] In addition to pulmonary veins, other sites, such as the posterior left atrium, ligament of Marshall, coronary sinus, venae cavae, septum, and appendages, serve as foci for AF.[3]

Warfarin Efficacy, Safety, and Limitations

Vitamin K antagonists (VKAs) have been the cornerstone of therapy for stroke prevention in AF. The anticoagulant effect of warfarin is measured by the international normalized ratio (INR). Based on stroke prevention trials in AF and cohort studies, the recommended INR range for prevention of stroke in patients with NVAF has been established to be 2.0 to 3.0.[12] A decrease in INR from 2.0 to 1.7 was previously shown to double the risk of ischemic stroke, and a further decrease to 1.4 further doubled the risk yet again.[12] An INR greater than 4 is associated with increased risk of subdural hemorrhage.[13]

The proportion of time spent in the INR range of 2.0 to 3.0, or time in therapeutic range (TTR), has been validated as a marker to predict outcomes of anticoagulation. Based on the post hoc analysis of the Atrial Fibrillation Clopidogrel Trial With Irbesartan for Prevention of Vascular Events (ACTIVE W) trial, a target threshold of TTR of at least 58% to 65% was necessary to demonstrate a benefit of warfarin over dual antiplatelet therapy in stroke prevention in AF.[14]

Nonetheless, there are numerous limitations to TTR. First, as TTR is a measure of anticoagulation over time, transient fluctuations in INR are not reflected by TTR; thus, risk of stroke or hemorrhage during these periods is difficult to assess.[12] Second, TTR is valid when INR is measured over consecutive periods of time; when there are gaps of more than 56 days, TTR is no longer accurate.[15]

Because warfarin has a narrow therapeutic range and there is great variation in daily dose requirements based on patients' characteristics, there is a risk of overanticoagulation and underanticoagulation. Given the difficulty in predicting the level of anticoagulation when initiating therapy with warfarin, genotype-guided dosing has also been studied. Polymorphisms in genes CYP2C9 and VKORC1, along with body surface area and age, have been shown to account for more than 50% variability in dosing. In the 455-subject prospective multicenter, randomized controlled trial, pharmacogenetic-based dosing versus control was associated with higher mean percentage of TTR (67.4% vs 60.3% adjusted difference, 7.0% points; 95% confidence interval [CI], 3.3–10.6) with fewer incidences of excessive anticoagulation and decreased time needed to reach therapeutic INR (21 vs 29 day [$P<.001$]).[16] Furthermore, a subgroup analysis of the Effective Anticoagulation with Factor Xa Next Generation in Atrial Fibrillation–Thrombolysis in Myocardial Infarction 48 (ENGAGE-AF TIMI 48) trial showed that patients with CYP2C9 and VKORC1 genotypes who corresponded to US Food and Drug Administration (FDA) categories of *sensitive* and *highly sensitive* responders to warfarin were more likely to be overanticoagulated and had higher rates of bleeding in the first 90 days of initiating treatment. Edoxaban, compared with warfarin, was associated with significantly less bleeding events, including fatal, life-threatening, intracranial, and major bleeding.[17] Although these results are promising, genotyping before warfarin prescription is not recommended given the lack of sufficient randomized controlled trial data, relatively brief window of utility, and uncertain cost-benefit.

Furthermore, other patient-specific factors that influence INR include nonwhite race, female sex, poverty, greater distance from care, active cancer, frequent hospitalizations, chronic liver disease, substance abuse, dementia, and major depression.[12,15]

Although there is more than 60 years of experience with warfarin as the only oral anticoagulant option, there are numerous limitations associated with its use. Warfarin has slow onset and offset of action, which is associated with long hospital stays and long periods of time to reach homeostasis. Furthermore, there are genetic variations in warfarin metabolism as well as numerous food and drug interactions, which make it difficult to achieve therapeutic levels of anticoagulation.[18]

Non–Vitamin K Antagonist Oral Anticoagulants (NOACs)

The many disadvantages of warfarin led to the development of NOACs. The predictable anticoagulant activity, short half-life, and minimal drug-drug interactions make NOACs a favorable alternative to warfarin. As is discussed further, the pivotal trials that compared NOACs with warfarin proved the comparable efficacy of NOACs in reducing the risks of stroke and thromboembolism and superior safety profile in reducing the risk of bleeding and mortality.

There are 4 NOACs currently approved in the United States, Europe, and Asia. They are dabigatran, rivaroxaban, apixaban, and edoxaban. Dabigatran was approved by the US FDA for prevention of stroke in patients with NVAF in 2010,[19] followed by rivaroxaban (2011),[20] apixaban (2012),[21] and most recently edoxaban (2015)[22] (**Table 3**).

Dabigatran

Dabigatran (Pradaxa) is a direct thrombin inhibitor, blocking the free- and clot-bound thrombin and thrombin-induced platelet aggregation (**Fig. 2**).[19] Its bioavailability is 3% to 7% and reaches peak plasma concentration in 1 to 2 hours after ingestion. The half-life of dabigatran ranges from 12 to 17 hours in patients with normal and mildly impaired renal function. However, because 80% is cleared renally, the half-life is longer in patients with severe renal insufficiency (**Table 1**).

Based on a large, randomized, open-label trial, Randomized Evaluation of Long-Term Anticoagulation Therapy (RE-LY),[23] 2 doses of dabigatran were approved for stroke prevention in patients with NVAF: 150 milligram (mg) and 75 mg; both are dosed orally twice daily. Although the 150-mg and 110-mg doses of dabigatran were studied in RE-LY, only the 150-mg dose was approved by the FDA. Both doses were noninferior to warfarin in preventing stroke and systemic embolic events (SEE); however, the

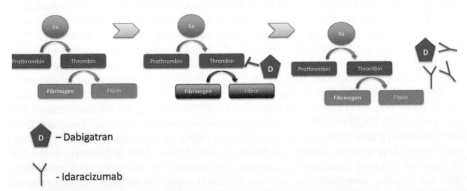

D – Dabigatran

Y - Idaracizumab

Fig. 2. Coagulation cascade and direct thrombin inhibitor target. Final common pathway of the coagulation cascade is shown. Dabigatran target in the cascade as well as mechanism of action of reversal agents is indicated.

Table 1
Properties of non–vitamin K antagonist oral anticoagulants

	Dabigatran	Rivaroxaban	Apixaban	Edoxaban
Trade name	Pradaxa	Xarelto	Eliquis	Savaysa (United States) Lixiana (other countries)
Target	Thrombin	Factor Xa	Factor Xa	Factor Xa
Half-life (h)	12–17	5–9 11–13 (in elderly)	12	10–14
Peak plasma concentration (h)	1	2–4	3–4	1–2
Renal clearance (%)	80	33	27	50
Protein binding (%)	35	>90	87	55

Data from Refs.[19–22]

150-mg dose was superior to warfarin in terms of efficacy, and the 110-mg dose was associated with significantly fewer bleeding events than warfarin. The 150-mg dose reduced the risk of stroke and SEE more than the 110-mg dose but also caused more bleeding. Subgroup analyses in more vulnerable patients (patients >75 years of age and those with moderate renal impairment [creatinine clearance (CrCL) 30–50 mL/min]) further confirmed these findings. Given that the irreversible sequelae of stroke is more clinically significant than nonfatal bleeding and the risk of undertreating with a lower dose would be associated with more strokes, the higher dose of dabigatran was favored.[24]

In the United States, the FDA approved the use of 75 mg dose based on pharmacokinetic and pharmacodynamic data in patients with a calculated CrCl of 15 to 30 mL/min.[19] The 75-mg dose should also be considered in patients with CrCl 30 to 50 mL/min who are taking a concomitant P-glycoprotein inhibitor. Outside the United States, the approved doses are 150 mg and 110 mg, with the lower dose preferred in patients at increased risk of bleeding, such as elderly patients and those with moderate renal dysfunction (**Table 2**).

In RE-LY, 18,113 patients with NVAF were randomized to receive dabigatran versus warfarin. The rates of stroke and SEE in the group that received the 150-mg dose of dabigatran twice daily were 1.11%/y versus 1.69%/y in the warfarin group (relative risk, 0.66; 95% CI, 0.53–0.82; P<.001 for superiority). The rates of major bleeding were 3.11%/y and 3.36%/y, respectively (P = .31). Additional important secondary findings from the RE-LY trial are summarized in **Table 3**.

The Long-term Multicenter Extension of Dabigatran Treatment in Patients with Atrial Fibrillation (RELY-ABLE) registry enrolled patients who had completed participation in the RE-LY clinical trial on the study drug and then followed these patients on extended therapy for an additional 2.3 years (median). During this continued treatment period, there were similar rates of stroke and SEE in the 150-mg and 110-mg doses of dabigatran with higher rates of major bleeding with the 150-mg dose. The rates of hemorrhagic stroke and intracranial bleeding remained low in the dabigatran group, consistent with findings in RE-LY.[25] Based on recent post-marketing surveillance data, which included 134,414 patients and 37,587 person-years of follow-up, the rates of stroke and SEE were similar among patients taking dabigatran versus warfarin with significantly fewer rates of intracranial hemorrhage (ICH). The rates of major bleeding were higher in the dabigatran group but did not reach significance.[26]

Table 2
Trials of non–vitamin K antagonist oral anticoagulants in atrial fibrillation

NOAC	Dabigatran	Rivaroxaban	Apixaban	Edoxaban
Trial name	RE-LY	ROCKET-AF	ARISTOTLE	ENGAGE AF-TIMI 48
US FDA–approved dosing	For CrCl >30 mL/min: 150 mg BID For CrCl 15–30 mL/min: 75 mg BID	For CrCl >50 mL/min: 20 mg Qd with evening meal For CrCl 15–50 mL/min: 15 mg Qd with the evening meal	5 mg BID In patients with at least 2 of the following: age ≥80 y, body weight ≤60 kg, or creatinine ≥1.5 mg/dL: 2.5 mg BID	For CrCl >50 to ≤95 mL/min: 60 mg Qd For CrCl 15–50 mL/min: reduce dose to 30 mg Qd For CrCl >95 mL/min: avoid use
Drug interactions	Avoid concomitant use with P-gp inducers For CrCl 30–50 mL/min and concomitant P-gp inhibitor[a] reduce dose to 75 mg BID For CrCl 15–30 mL/min avoid concomitant use with P-gp inhibitors	Avoid concomitant use with combined P-gp and strong CYP3A4 inhibitors[b] or moderate CYP3A4 inhibitor[c] Avoid concomitant use of combined P-gp and strong CYP3A4 inducers[d] For patients taking 2.5 mg BID dose, avoid concomitant use with strong dual inhibitors of CYP3A4 and P-gp	Decrease dose by 50% if concomitant use with strong dual inhibitors of CYP3A4 and P-gp[e]	Avoid use with rifampin

Abbreviations: ARISTOTLE, Apixaban for Reduction in Stroke and Other Thromboembolic Events in Atrial Fibrillation; BID, twice daily; CrCl, creatinine clearance; CYP, cytochrome P450; ENGAGE AF-TIMI 48, Effective Anticoagulation with Factor Xa Next Generation in Atrial Fibrillation–Thrombolysis in Myocardial Infarction Study 48; FDA, Food and Drug Administration; NOAC, Non–Vitamin K oral anticoagulant; P-gp, permeability glycoprotein; Qd, once daily; RE-LY, Randomized Evaluation of Long-term Anticoagulation Therapy; ROCKET-AF, Rivaroxaban Once Daily Oral Direct Factor Xa inhibition compared with vitamin K antagonism for prevention of stroke and embolism trial in atrial fibrillation.

[a] Dronedarone or systemic ketoconazole.
[b] Ketoconazole, ritonavir, clarithromycin, and erythromycin.
[c] Fluconazole.
[d] Carbamazepine, phenytoin, rifampin, St. John's wort.
[e] Ketoconazole, itraconazole, ritonavir, or clarithromycin.

Table 3
Key findings from the non–vitamin K antagonist oral anticoagulant trials in atrial fibrillation

Trial	RE-LY		ROCKET-AF	ARISTOTLE	ENGAGE-AF TIMI 48	
NOAC	Dabigatran 110 mg vs VKA	Dabigatran 150 mg vs VKA	Rivaroxaban vs VKA	Apixaban vs VKA	Edoxaban 60/30 mg vs VKA	Edoxaban 30/15 mg vs VKA
Primary end point (stroke, SEE), HR (CI), _P_ value for non-inferiority						
	0.91 (0.74–1.11) $P<.001$	0.66 (0.53–0.82) $P<.001$	0.88 (0.75–1.03)[b] $P<.001$	0.79 (0.66–0.95) $P<.001$	0.79 (0.63–0.99)[a] $P<.001$	1.07 (0.87–1.31) $P = .005$
Principal safety outcome, HR (CI), _P_ value						
	0.8 (0.69–0.93) $P = .003$	0.93 (0.81–1.07) $P = .31$	1.03 (0.96–1.11) $P = .44$	0.69 (0.60–0.80) $P<.001$	0.8 (0.71–0.91) $P<.001$	0.47 (0.41–0.55) $P<.001$
Death any cause, HR (CI), _P_ value						
	0.91 (0.8–1.01) $P = .13$	0.88 (0.77–1.00) $P = .051$	0.71 (0.49–1.03) $P = .075$	0.89 (0.80–0.998) $P = .047$	0.92 (0.83–1.01) $P = .08$	0.87 (0.79–0.96) $P = .006$
GI bleed, HR (CI), _P_ value						
	1.1 (0.86–1.41) $P = .43$	1.5 (1.19–1.89) $P<.001$	1.34; $P<.0001$	0.89 (0.7–1.15) $P = .37$	1.23 (1.02–1.50) $P = .03$	0.67 (0.53–0.83) $P<.001$
Myocardial infarction HR (CI), _P_ value						
	1.35 (0.98–1.87) $P = .07$	1.38 (1.00–1.91) $P = .048$	0.81 (0.63–1.06) $P = .121$	0.88 (0.66–1.17) $P = .37$	0.94 (0.74–1.19) $P = .6$	1.19 (0.95–1.49) $P = .13$

Abbreviations: GI, gastrointestinal; HR, hazard ratio; SEE, systemic embolic event.
[a] Modified intention to treat population.
[b] Intention to treat population.

Rivaroxaban

Rivaroxaban (Xarelto) is a direct factor Xa (FXa) and prothrombinase-bound FXa inhibitor (**Fig. 3**).[20] Its bioavailability is dose dependent; for the 15-mg and-20 mg doses, bioavailability increases with concomitant food intake. Rivaroxaban reaches peak plasma concentration in 2 to 4 hours. Approximately 66% of a rivaroxaban dose is eliminated via kidneys; renal metabolism accounts for 33% of its clearance, and the other 33% is excreted in urine unchanged (**Table 1**).[27]

There are 2 doses of rivaroxaban approved in the United States for stroke prevention in patients with NVAF: 15 mg and 20 mg. The recommended dose is 20 mg administered orally once daily with meals for CrCl greater than 50 mL/min with the dose reduced to 15 mg once daily for CrCl 15 to 50 mL/min.[20] Concomitant use of rivaroxaban and strong permeability glycoprotein (P-gp) inhibitors/inducers and CYP3A4 inhibitors/inducers should be avoided (**Table 2**).

Based on a large, double-blind trial, Rivaroxaban Once-Daily Oral Direct Factor Xa Inhibition Compared with Vitamin K Antagonism for Prevention of Stroke and Embolism Trial in Atrial Fibrillation (ROCKET AF), rivaroxaban was approved for stroke prevention in patients with NVAF. In the ROCKET AF trial, 14,264 patients were randomized to receive rivaroxaban versus warfarin. The rates of stroke or SEE were 1.7%/y versus 2.2%/y in the experimental and control groups, respectively (hazard ratio [HR], 0.79; 95% CI, 0.66–0.96; $P<.001$ for noninferiority).[28] Furthermore, the rates of

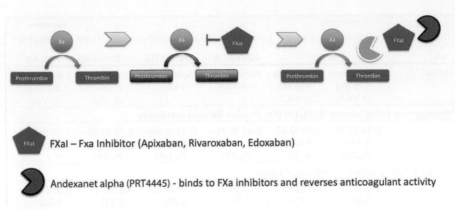

FXaI – Fxa Inhibitor (Apixaban, Rivaroxaban, Edoxaban)

Andexanet alpha (PRT4445) - binds to FXa inhibitors and reverses anticoagulant activity

Ciraparntag (aripazine, PER977) – binds to FXa inhibitors and reverses anticoagulant activity

Fig. 3. Coagulation cascade and FXa inhibitor targets. Final common pathway of the coagulation cascade is shown. FXa inhibitor targets in the cascade are shown, and mechanism of action of reversal agents is indicated.

major and nonmajor clinically relevant bleeding were similar across patients receiving rivaroxaban and warfarin (14.9%/y and 14.5%/y, respectively; HR, 1.03; 95% CI, 0.96–1.11; $P = .44$).[28] Key secondary findings from ROCKET AF are summarized in **Table 3**.

Apixaban

Apixaban (Eliquis) is a free- and clot-bound FXa and prothrombinase-complex inhibitor (see **Fig. 3**). Its bioavailability is 50% and is not affected by concomitant food intake. It reaches peak plasma concentration in 3 to 4 hours and is eliminated in urine and feces, with urine clearance accounting for 27% of total clearance (**Table 1**).[21]

There are 2 doses of apixaban available in the United States: 2.5 mg and 5.0 mg dosed orally twice daily. For stroke prevention in patients with NVAF, the recommended dosage is 5.0 mg administered orally twice daily with dose reduction to 2.5 mg twice daily in patients with any 2 of the following: 80 years of age or older, body weight of 60 kg or less, or serum creatinine of 1.5 mg/dL or greater.[21] Dose reduction by 50% is recommended when coadministering a 5-mg dose of apixaban with strong inhibitors of cytochrome P450 3A4 (CYP3A4) and P-gp. Concomitant use of apixaban (at any dose) with strong dual inhibitors of CYP3A4 and P-gp is not recommended (**Table 2**).[21]

Based on a large double-blind trial, Apixaban for Reduction in Stroke and Other Thromboembolic Events in Atrial Fibrillation (ARISTOTLE), apixaban was approved for stroke prevention in patients with NVAF. In ARISTOTLE, 18, 201 patients with NVAF were randomized to receive apixaban versus warfarin. The rates of stroke or SEE in apixaban and warfarin groups were 1.27%/y and 1.60%/y, respectively (HR, 0.79; 95% CI, 0.66–0.95; $P = .01$ for superiority).[29] Patients who received apixaban also had lower rates of bleeding compared with warfarin (2.13%/y and 3.09%/y, respectively; HR, 0.69; 95% CI, 0.60–0.80; $P<.001$).[29] Additional key findings from ARISTOTLE are summarized in **Table 3**.

Apixaban was compared with aspirin in patients who were not willing or able to take a VKA in a double-blind randomized trial known as Apixaban Versus Acetylsalicylic Acid to Prevent Stroke in Atrial Fibrillation Patients Who Have Failed or Are Unsuitable for Vitamin K Antagonist Treatment (AVERROES). The trial enrolled 5599 patients with AF and increased risk of stroke, who were treated with either apixaban 5 mg twice daily versus aspirin 81 to 324 mg once daily. The trial was terminated early as clear benefit of apixaban over aspirin was seen in preventing stroke and SEE with similar rates of bleeding.[30]

Edoxaban

Edoxaban (Savaysa in the United States, Lixiana outside the United States) is an FXa inhibitor with greater than 10,000-fold increased affinity to FXa than thrombin (see **Fig. 3**).[31] Its bioavailability is 62%, and it reaches peak plasma concentration in 1 to 2 hours. It has dual renal (50%) and extrarenal clearance (**Table 1**).[19,32]

There are 3 available doses approved in the United States: 15 mg, 30 mg, and 60 mg dosed orally once daily. For stroke prevention in patients with NVAF, the recommended dosage is 60 mg once daily in patients with CrCL greater than 50 to 95 mL/min or less. Dose reduction is recommended in patients with CrCl 15 to 50 mL/min, whereas edoxaban is not recommended in those with CrCl greater than 95 mL/min.[19] The US FDA recommends no dose reduction with concomitant P-gp inhibitor use, but coadministration with potent P-gp inducers should be avoided. Outside the United States, most regulatory authorities recommend a 50% dose reduction when concomitant strong P-gp inhibitors are used (eg, dronedarone, verapamil, quinidine), and for body weight ≤ 60 kg, with no limitation for use for CrCL >95 mL/min. When transitioning from 60 mg edoxaban to VKA, the 30-mg edoxaban dose is started concomitantly with warfarin until therapeutic INR is reached. When transitioning from 30 mg edoxaban to VKA, the 15-mg edoxaban dose is used instead (**Table 2**).

Based on the largest and longest randomized trial of a NOAC, the ENGAGE AF-TIMI 48 trial, edoxaban was approved for stroke prevention in patients with NVAF. In the ENGAGE AF-TIMI 48 trial 21,105 patients were randomized to receive a higher-dose edoxaban regimen (60 mg with dose reduction to 30 mg), lower-dose edoxaban regimen (30 mg with dose reduction to 15 mg), or warfarin in a double-blind, double-dummy fashion. The rates of stroke and SEE were 1.18%/y and 1.61%/y in the higher- and lower-dose groups of edoxaban, compared with warfarin 1.50%/y (HR, 0.79; 97.5% CI, 0.63–0.99; $P<.001$ for noninferiority and HR, 1.07; 97.5% CI, 0.87–1.31; $P = .005$ for noninferiority, respectively). The rates of major bleeding were 2.75%/y and 1.61%/y in the higher- and lower-dose groups of edoxaban, compared with warfarin 3.43%/y (HR, 0.80; 95% CI, 0.71–0.91; $P<.001$ for noninferiority and HR, 0.47; 95% CI, 0.41–0.55; $P<.001$ for noninferiority, respectively).[33] Other findings from ENGAGE AF-TIMI 48 are summarized in **Table 3**.

NON–VITAMIN K ANTAGONIST ORAL ANTICOAGULANTS
Specific Patient Scenarios and Populations

Mechanical heart valves

Following the approval of dabigatran for stroke prevention in NVAF, a phase II dose validation study to Evaluate the Safety and Pharmacokinetics of Oral Dabigatran Etexilate in Patients after Heart Valve Replacement (RE-ALIGN)[34] was conducted to study the use of dabigatran in mechanical heart valves. Two patient populations were studied: those who had undergone aortic or mitral valve replacements within the past 7 days or past 3 months. Patients were randomized in a 2:1 ratio to receive dabigatran (dose adjusted based on renal function to achieve rough plasma level of at least 50 ng/mL) or warfarin (INR goal 2–3 or 2.5–3.5 based on thromboembolic risk). The study was terminated early, as dabigatran was associated with an increased risk of thromboembolic and bleeding events as compared with warfarin. Most of the thromboembolic events were seen in patients who underwent mechanical valve implantation within 7 days of initiation of dabigatran. The rapid onset of dabigatran versus warfarin may account for the increased bleeding rates in the directly postoperative patient population versus the group that received the drug after 3 months of operation.[35] Furthermore, the increased thromboembolic events in the experimental group may be explained by a prothrombotic postoperative state and subtherapeutic dabigatran plasma levels. It should also be noted that the 50 ng/mL cutoff was based on data from the RE-LY trial, which studied the drug for another indication.[35] Based on RE-ALIGN, currently NOACs are not recommended for anticoagulation in patients with mechanical heart valves, despite the absence of data with FXa inhibitors.

Cardioversion

Data regarding the efficacy and safety of NOACs in patients undergoing cardioversion come from post hoc analyses of the large warfarin-controlled phase 3 trials of NOACs and one medium-sized prospective randomized study.

A retrospective analysis of the RE-LY trial[36] demonstrated that the rates of stroke and SEE as well as major bleeding after cardioversion were low and comparable in the dabigatran and warfarin groups suggesting that dabigatran could be used in the setting of cardioversion. With that said, the study was not powered to show a difference among the 3 arms it compared (2 doses of dabigatran and warfarin) given the low rates of events.[36]

Similar post hoc analyses were conducted on the data from ROCKET-AF, showing no significant differences in stroke or SEE (HR 1.38; 95% CI 0.61–3.11; $P = .44$) and death (HR 1.57; 95% CI 0.69–3.55; $P = .28$) following cardioversion or AF ablation in patients treated with rivaroxaban versus warfarin.[37] There was an increase in hospitalization seen after the procedure (HR 2.01; 95% CI 1.51–2.68; $P<.0001$). In the post hoc analysis[38] of data from the ARISTOTLE trial, there were no events of stroke or SEE in all patients who underwent cardioversion, whereas the rates of major bleeding and death were comparable. Similar results with edoxaban were recently reported.[39]

In the Explore the Efficacy and Safety of Once-daily Oral Rivaroxaban for the Prevention of Cardiovascular Events in Subjects with Nonvalvular Atrial Fibrillation Scheduled for Cardioversion (XVERT) trial, 1504 patients were randomized to receive either open-label rivaroxaban or warfarin before elective cardioversion. Patients were further subdivided into early (1–5 days) and late (3–8 weeks) planned cardioversion groups. Thromboembolic and bleeding events were noted to be similar in the rivaroxaban and warfarin groups, and this also applied to the early and late cardioversion strategies. Furthermore, in the delayed cardioversion group, rivaroxaban was associated with shorter time to cardioversion than warfarin, as it took longer periods of time to achieve therapeutic INR.[40]

Chronic kidney disease

Data are sparse regarding the use of NOACs in patients with NVAF and severe (stage IV) or end-stage chronic kidney disease, as each of the large phase 3 trials excluded patients with CrCl less than 25 to 30 mL/min. In the United States, dabigatran, rivaroxaban, and edoxaban are not recommended for use in patients with CrCl less than 15 mL/min, whereas the apixaban label does permit use in patients with end-stage renal disease on stable hemodialysis based on pharmacokinetic modeling, as it is the NOAC with the least renal clearance.

In a subgroup analysis of the RE-LY trial, the efficacy of dabigatran was consistent across all levels of renal impairment. Furthermore, rates of stroke or systemic embolism, all-cause death, and major bleeding increased with worsening renal function.[41]

Population pharmacokinetic and pharmacodynamic analyses from the ROCKET-AF trial showed that a reduced dose of rivaroxaban of 15 mg in patients with moderate renal impairment (CrCl 30–49 mL/min) had similar drug exposures as the standard dose of 20 mg in patients with normal or mildly reduced renal function.[42]

In the largest subgroup analysis of the ARISTOTLE trial based on renal impairment,[43] safety and efficacy of apixaban versus warfarin was studied in 7587 patients with an estimated glomerular filtration rate (eGFR) of greater than 50 to 80 mL/min and 3017 patients with an eGFR of 50 mL/min or less. Consistent with prior studies, decreasing renal function was associated with increased risk of stroke. However, primary end points of stroke and SEE occurred less in patients receiving apixaban regardless of renal impairment. The rates of major bleeding were also less frequent in the apixaban group across all levels of renal impairment.

In a unique aspect to the study design, the ENGAGE AF-TIMI 48 protocol allowed for dynamic dose adjustment of the study drug during the trial to account for changing renal function, body weight, and drug interactions that occurred after randomization. Subgroup analysis of patients who received the 50% dose reduction of edoxaban because of CrCl of 50 mL/min or less, weight of 60 kg or less, or potent P-gp inhibitor use showed that efficacy was preserved with even greater reduction in bleeding events when compared with warfarin.[33] The US FDA recommends that patients with CrCl 15 to 50 mL/min receive edoxaban 30 mg instead of 60 mg. In patients with CrCl greater than 95 mL/min, edoxaban blood levels are 40% lower than in patients with CrCl of greater than 50 to 80 mL/min or less; in the former subgroup, the rates of ischemic stroke were higher when compared with warfarin (HR [95% CI]: 2.16 [1.17, 3.97]) with lower rates of bleeding. Thus, the US FDA recommends a different anticoagulant other than edoxaban be used in patients with AF and CrCl greater than 95 mL/min.[22] Of note, this restriction does not apply in the United States to patients with venothromboembolism; regulatory authorities in Europe and Asia did not issue such a restriction on the use of edoxaban in patients with higher CrCl.

Measuring Anticoagulation

One of the advantages of NOACs is the lack of need of routine monitoring of anticoagulation. However, in special circumstances, such as severe bleeding and before emergent surgical procedures, it may be desirable to assess the degree of anticoagulation.[43,44,45] Currently there are no FDA-approved NOAC assays; but the diluted thrombin time (dTT), activated partial thromboplastin time (aPTT), ecarin clotting time (ECT), and chromogenic anti-Xa assay for FXa inhibitors have been explored and may be helpful in selected situations.[46]

The aPTT prolongs in a curvilinear relationship with dose of dabigatran[47] but achieves such high levels at higher concentrations of dabigatran that it becomes unreliable for clinical use in this range.[48] Furthermore, sensitivity and specificity of the assay depends on the type of reagent used. Levels of aPTT greater than 2 times the upper limit of normal have been shown to correlate with increased bleeding risk. Prothrombin time (PT)/INR was shown to be less sensitive than aPTT and depends strongly on the type of reagent and whether a hospital/laboratory-based INR measurement was used versus a point-of-care–based method.[48] ECT is prolonged linearly in a concentration-dependent manner, and levels greater than 3 times the upper limit of normal have been shown to correlate with increased bleeding.[44,47] Thrombin time assays have been shown to be overly sensitive, but use of dTT assays can overcome this limitation. Although dabigatran causes a concentration-dependent prolongation of dTT, the assay is not widely available.[48]

For the oral FXa inhibitors, the INR is not a reliable method to measure the level of anticoagulation. FXa inhibitors prolong PT in a concentration-dependent manner; however, the effect on PT depends on type of FXa inhibitor, time of last ingestion of FXa, and type of reagent used.[44] aPTT assays have been shown to have unacceptably low sensitivity.[48] Chromogenic anti-FXa assays are a promising alternative, as they have been shown to have a linear and concentration-dependent relationship in apixaban and rivaroxaban trials when calibrated with low-molecular-weight heparin standards.[48]

Managing Bleeding

Both the American College of Cardiology (ACC), through the College's Anticoagulation Initiative,[49] and the European Heart Rhythm Association (EHRA)[50] recently published expert recommendations on management of interruption of NOACs, bleeding, and reversal of the anticoagulant effect.

In case of bleeding, the initial assessment should include determination of onset, site, volume, and rate of bleeding. The time of last ingestion of NOAC should be determined, concomitant medications reviewed, and anticoagulant and antiplatelet agents held. Next, basic laboratory work including complete blood count, PT, activated thromboplastin time, and renal and hepatic function panels should be reviewed.[49] It is important to note that because the half-life of NOACs is short, in cases of minor bleeding, usually just holding the dose of NOAC and supportive measures with fluids, red cell transfusion, and mechanical compression (if feasible) are adequate to achieve hemostasis.[45] Depending on timing of NOAC ingestion (ie, if within 6 hours), gastric lavage or oral charcoal may be considered.[51] Furthermore, hemodialysis is an option for management of bleeding in case of dabigatran because of its low protein binding; however, hemodialysis is not an option with FXa inhibitors as they are highly protein bound.[49]

In cases whereby the bleeding site can be identified, endoscopic and surgical procedures may be necessary. Vitamin K does not reverse the anticoagulant effects of NOACs, and physiologic quantities of fresh frozen plasma do not supply enough quantities of FXa and thrombin; given that NOACs work by blocking FXa and thrombin, transfusing plasma will not be effective.[45]

Prothrombin complex concentrates (PCCs) represent another therapy that has been studied. PCCs come in 3-factor concentrates (containing factors II, IX, and X), 4-factor concentrates (also containing factor VII), activated prothrombin concentrates (containing activated forms of these factors), and some formulations that include proteins C and S.[45] The PCCs have been shown to have mixed results in reversing NOACs.[52,53] Thus, risks of prothrombotic events must be weighed against anticoagulant benefits.[49] Based on guidelines from the EHRA and ACC, administration of PCC and aPCC may be considered in cases of life-threatening bleeding, though data from registries have shown that this is rarely necessary.[49]

With regard to restarting anticoagulation, benefits of bleeding must be weighed with risks of holding anticoagulation. In cases of minor gastrointestinal (GI) bleeds, switching to apixaban or edoxaban 30 mg may be an option as risk of GI bleed is less frequent with these agents. Others may benefit from a switch to VKA, which has a lower rate of GI bleeding than rivaroxaban and higher dose regimens of dabigatran and edoxaban.[48]

Reversal Agents

In October 2015, the FDA approved the use of idarucizumab, a humanized monoclonal antibody fragment that specifically binds to dabigatran and prevents its binding to factor IIa. In the Reversal Effects of Idarucizumab on Active Dabigatran (RE-VERSE AD) trial,[49] idarucizumab was administered to 90 patients taking dabigatran who had either serious bleeding or required an urgent procedure. Within minutes of administration of idarucizumab, concentrations of unbound dabigatran were detected to be less than 20 ng/mL, a level that has no anticoagulant effect, in all but 1 patient. Idarucizumab reversed anticoagulant activity in 88% to 98% patients with median maximum reversal of 100% (95% CI 100%–100%). Normal intraoperative hemostasis was achieved in 92% of patients undergoing an urgent procedure, and only 1 thrombotic event was observed after administration of study drug.

Currently there are no reversal agents for FXa inhibitors that are available for clinical use, although 2 are in late-stage development. (Andexanet alpha (PRT4445)[54] is a "decoy FXa" that binds to FXa inhibitors in the blood and prevents their interaction with FXa. Several phase 3 trials have demonstrated the ability of Andexanet alpha to reverse the anticoagulant effect of rivaroxaban and apixiban.[55] PER977 (known as ciraparantag in the United States and aripazine in Europe) is another reversal agent that can be used to reverse the anticoagulant effect of inhibitors of factor IIa and FXa (including both oral and parenteral anticoagulants) and is being developed by Perosphere.[55,56]

Summary

The comparable efficacy of NOACs to warfarin in preventing stroke and SEE and superior safety profile in decreasing rates of ICH and mortality have led to worldwide use of these agents. Availability of multiple dosing regimens and favorable subanalyses and postsurveillance data in special populations, such as elderly, those with renal impairment, and patients undergoing cardioversion, further demonstrate the versatility of these agents. Lastly, with increasing experience with NOACs, expert recommendations on management of bleeding are now available; with promising results, multiple reversal agents are in the late stages of drug development.

POST ACCEPTANCE UPDATE

After the acceptance of this manuscript, the results of the ENSURE-AF (Edoxaban vs. Warfarin in Subjects Undergoing Cardioversion of Atrial Fibrillation) were published (Goette A, Merino JL, Ezekowitz MD, et al, Lancet Published online August 30, 2016 http://dx.doi.org/10.1016/S0140-6736(16)31474-X). In this open-label randomized controlled trial of 2199 patients with atrial fibrillation undergoing electrical cardioversion for atrial fibrillation, edoxaban was compared to enoxaparin-warfarin. The primary efficacy composite of stroke, systemic embolism, myocardial infarction, or cardiovascular death occurred in 5 (0.46%) of patients randomized to edoxaban vs 11 patients (1.0%) in the enoxaparin-warfarin group (OR 0.46, 95% CI 0.12-1.43). There was no difference in the primary safety endpoint of major and clinically relevant non-major bleeding (1.5% vs 1.0%, OR 1.48, 95% CI 0.64-3.55). The results were independent of whether transesophageal echocardiography had been performed and the patients anticoagulant status (naïve vs experienced) prior to the study.

REFERENCES

1. McManus DD, Rienstra M, Benjamin EJ. An update on the prognosis of patients with atrial fibrillation. Circulation 2012;126(10):e143–6.
2. Go AS, Hylek EM, Phillips KA, et al. Prevalence of diagnosed atrial fibrillation in adults: national implications for rhythm management and stroke prevention: the

Anticoagulation and Risk Factors in Atrial Fibrillation (ATRIA) Study. JAMA 2001; 285(18):2370–5.

3. January CT, Wann LS, Alpert JS, et al. 2014 AHA/ACC/HRS guideline for the management of patients with atrial fibrillation: a report of the American College of Cardiology/American Heart Association Task Force on Practice Guidelines and the Heart Rhythm Society. J Am Coll Cardiol 2014;64(21):e1–76.

4. Kim MH, Johnston SS, Chu BC, et al. Estimation of total incremental health care costs in patients with atrial fibrillation in the United States. Circ Cardiovasc Qual Outcomes 2011;4(3):313–20.

5. Nabauer M, Gerth A, Limbourg T, et al. The Registry of the German Competence NETwork on atrial fibrillation: patient characteristics and initial management. Europace 2009;11(4):423–34.

6. Nerheim P, Birger-Botkin S, Piracha L, et al. Heart failure and sudden death in patients with tachycardia-induced cardiomyopathy and recurrent tachycardia. Circulation 2004;110(3):247–52.

7. De Caterina R, Camm AJ. What is 'valvular' atrial fibrillation? A reappraisal. Eur Heart J 2014;35(47):3328–35.

8. Watson T, Shantsila E, Lip GY. Mechanisms of thrombogenesis in atrial fibrillation: Virchow's triad revisited. Lancet 2009;373(9658):155–66.

9. Tucker NR, Ellinor PT. Emerging directions in the genetics of atrial fibrillation. Circ Res 2014;114(9):1469–82.

10. Neelankavil J, Rau CD, Wang Y. The genetic basis of coronary artery disease and atrial fibrillation: a search for disease mechanisms and therapeutic targets. J Cardiothorac Vasc Anesth 2015;29(5):1328–32.

11. Ehrlich JR, Cha TJ, Zhang L, et al. Cellular electrophysiology of canine pulmonary vein cardiomyocytes: action potential and ionic current properties. J Physiol 2003;551(Pt 3):801–13.

12. Hylek EM, Skates SJ, Sheehan MA, et al. An analysis of the lowest effective intensity of prophylactic anticoagulation for patients with nonrheumatic atrial fibrillation. N Engl J Med 1996;335(8):540–6.

13. Hylek EM, Singer DE. Risk factors for intracranial hemorrhage in outpatients taking warfarin. Ann Intern Med 1994;120(11):897–902.

14. Connolly SJ, Pogue J, Eikelboom J, et al. Benefit of oral anticoagulant over antiplatelet therapy in atrial fibrillation depends on the quality of international normalized ratio control achieved by centers and countries as measured by time in therapeutic range. Circulation 2008;118(20):2029–37.

15. Rose AJ, Miller DR, Ozonoff A, et al. Gaps in monitoring during oral anticoagulation: insights into care transitions, monitoring barriers, and medication nonadherence. Chest 2013;143(3):751–7.

16. Pirmohamed M, Burnside G, Eriksson N, et al. A randomized trial of genotype-guided dosing of warfarin. N Engl J Med 2013;369(24):2294–303.

17. Mega JL, Walker JR, Ruff CT, et al. Genetics and the clinical response to warfarin and edoxaban: findings from the randomised, double-blind ENGAGE AF-TIMI 48 trial. Lancet 2015;385(9984):2280–7.

18. Ruff CT, Giugliano RP, Braunwald E, et al. New oral anticoagulants in patients with atrial fibrillation - Authors' reply. Lancet 2014;384(9937):25–6.

19. Pradaxa (Dabigatran Etexilate) [package insert]. Ridgefield, CT: Boehringer Ingelheim Pharmaceuticals; 2015.

20. Xaralto (Rivaroxaban) [package insert]. Titusville, FL: N.J.P. and I; 2015.

21. Eliquis (Apixaban) [package insert]. Princeton, NJ: Bristol-Myers Squibb; 2015.

22. Savaysa (Edoxaban) [package insert]. Tokyo: J.D.S; 2015.

23. Connolly SJ, Ezekowitz MD, Yusuf S, et al. Dabigatran versus warfarin in patients with atrial fibrillation. N Engl J Med 2009;361(12):1139–51.
24. Beasley BN, Unger EF, Temple R. Anticoagulant options–why the FDA approved a higher but not a lower dose of dabigatran. N Engl J Med 2011;364(19):1788–90.
25. Connolly SJ, Wallentin L, Ezekowitz MD, et al. The long-term multicenter observational study of Dabigatran treatment in patients with atrial fibrillation (RELY-ABLE) study. Circulation 2013;128(3):237–43.
26. Graham DJ, Reichman ME, Wernecke M, et al. Cardiovascular, bleeding, and mortality risks in elderly Medicare patients treated with dabigatran or warfarin for nonvalvular atrial fibrillation. Circulation 2015;131(2):157–64.
27. Weinz C, Schwarz T, Kubitza D, et al. Metabolism and excretion of rivaroxaban, an oral, direct factor Xa inhibitor, in rats, dogs, and humans. Drug Metab Dispos 2009;37(5):1056–64.
28. Patel MR, Mahaffey KW, Garg J, et al. Rivaroxaban versus warfarin in nonvalvular atrial fibrillation. N Engl J Med 2011;365(10):883–91.
29. Granger CB, Alexander JH, McMurray JJ, et al. Apixaban versus warfarin in patients with atrial fibrillation. N Engl J Med 2011;365(11):981–92.
30. Connolly SJ, Eikelboom J, Joyner C, et al. Apixaban in patients with atrial fibrillation. N Engl J Med 2011;364(9):806–17.
31. Furugohri T, Isobe K, Honda Y, et al. DU-176b, a potent and orally active factor Xa inhibitor: in vitro and in vivo pharmacological profiles. J Thromb Haemost 2008; 6(9):1542–9.
32. Gonzalez-Quesada CJ, Giugliano RP. Comparison of the phase III clinical trial designs of novel oral anticoagulants versus warfarin for the treatment of nonvalvular atrial fibrillation: implications for clinical practice. Am J Cardiovasc Drugs 2014; 14(2):111–27.
33. Giugliano RP, Ruff CT, Braunwald E, et al. Edoxaban versus warfarin in patients with atrial fibrillation. N Engl J Med 2013;369(22):2093–104.
34. Eikelboom JW, Connolly SJ, Brueckmann M, et al. Dabigatran versus warfarin in patients with mechanical heart valves. N Engl J Med 2013;369(13):1206–14.
35. Hylek EM. Dabigatran and mechanical heart valves–not as easy as we hoped. N Engl J Med 2013;369(13):1264–6.
36. Nagarakanti R, Ezekowitz MD, Oldgren J, et al. Dabigatran versus warfarin in patients with atrial fibrillation: an analysis of patients undergoing cardioversion. Circulation 2011;123(2):131–6.
37. Piccini JP, Stevens SR, Lokhnygina Y, et al. Outcomes after cardioversion and atrial fibrillation ablation in patients treated with rivaroxaban and warfarin in the ROCKET AF trial. J Am Coll Cardiol 2013;61(19):1998–2006.
38. Flaker G, Lopes RD, Al-Khatib SM, et al. Efficacy and safety of apixaban in patients after cardioversion for atrial fibrillation: insights from the ARISTOTLE trial (apixaban for reduction in stroke and other thromboembolic events in atrial fibrillation). J Am Coll Cardiol 2014;63(11):1082–7.
39. Plitt A, Ezekowitz MD, De Caterina R, et al. Cardioversion of atrial fibrillation in ENGAGE AF-TIMI 48. Clin Cardiol 2016;39(6):345–6.
40. Cappato R, Ezekowitz MD, Klein AL, et al. Rivaroxaban vs. vitamin K antagonists for cardioversion in atrial fibrillation. Eur Heart J 2014;35(47):3346–55.
41. Hijazi Z, Hohnloser SH, Oldgren J, et al. Efficacy and safety of dabigatran compared with warfarin in relation to baseline renal function in patients with atrial fibrillation: a RE-LY (randomized evaluation of long-term anticoagulation therapy) trial analysis. Circulation 2014;129(9):961–70.

42. Girgis IG, Patel MR, Peters GR, et al. Population pharmacokinetics and pharma-codynamics of rivaroxaban in patients with non-valvular atrial fibrillation: results from ROCKET AF. J Clin Pharmacol 2014;54(8):917–27.

43. Hohnloser SH, Hijazi Z, Thomas L, et al. Efficacy of apixaban when compared with warfarin in relation to renal function in patients with atrial fibrillation: insights from the ARISTOTLE trial. Eur Heart J 2012;33(22):2821–30.

44. Plitt A, Giugliano RP. Target-specific oral anticoagulants: practice issues for the clinician. Hosp Pract (1995) 2014;42(3):48–61.

45. Majeed A, Schulman S. Bleeding and antidotes in new oral anticoagulants. Best Pract Res Clin Haematol 2013;26(2):191–202.

46. Kalabalik J, Rattinger GB, Sullivan J, et al. Use of non-vitamin K antagonist oral anticoagulants in special patient populations with nonvalvular atrial fibrillation: a review of the literature and application to clinical practice. Drugs 2015;75(9): 979–98.

47. Stangier J, Rathgen K, Stähle H, et al. The pharmacokinetics, pharmacody-namics and tolerability of dabigatran etexilate, a new oral direct thrombin inhibi-tor, in healthy male subjects. Br J Clin Pharmacol 2007;64(3):292–303.

48. Cuker A, Siegal DM, Crowther MA, et al. Laboratory measurement of the antico-agulant activity of the non-vitamin K oral anticoagulants. J Am Coll Cardiol 2014; 64(11):1128–39.

49. Kovacs RJ, Flaker GC, Saxonhouse SJ, et al. Practical management of anticoa-gulation in patients with atrial fibrillation. J Am Coll Cardiol 2015;65(13):1340–60.

50. Heidbuchel H, Verhamme P, Alings M, et al. Updated European Heart Rhythm As-sociation practical guide on the use of non-vitamin K antagonist anticoagulants in patients with non-valvular atrial fibrillation. Europace 2015;17(10):1467–507.

51. van Ryn J, Stangier J, Haertter S, et al. Dabigatran etexilate–a novel, reversible, oral direct thrombin inhibitor: interpretation of coagulation assays and reversal of anticoagulant activity. Thromb Haemost 2010;103(6):1116–27.

52. Siegal DM, Cuker A. Reversal of novel oral anticoagulants in patients with major bleeding. J Thromb Thrombolysis 2013;35(3):391–8.

53. Dzik WH. Reversal of oral factor Xa inhibitors by prothrombin complex concen-trates: a re-appraisal. J Thromb Haemost 2015;13(Suppl 1):S187–94.

54. Enriquez A, Lip GY, Baranchuk A. Anticoagulation reversal in the era of the non-vitamin K oral anticoagulants. Europace 2015. [Epub ahead of print].

55. Siegal DM, Curnutte JT, Connolly SJ, et al. Andexanet Alfa for the reversal of Fac-tor Xa inhibitor activity. N Engl J Med 2015;373(25):2413–24.

56. Ansell JE, Bakhru SH, Laulicht BE, et al. Use of PER977 to reverse the anticoag-ulant effect of edoxaban. N Engl J Med 2014;371(22):2141–2.

Use of the Direct Oral Anticoagulants for the Treatment of Venous Thromboembolism

 CrossMark

Nicoletta Riva, MD, Walter Ageno, MD*

KEYWORDS

- Antithrombins • Factor Xa inhibitors • Pulmonary embolism • Venous thrombosis

KEY POINTS

- The direct oral anticoagulants have favorable pharmacologic profile: specific target on thrombin or factor Xa, rapid onset of action and short half-life, and predictable anticoagulant response.
- In the acute treatment of venous thromboembolism, they were noninferior in efficacy compared with the standard treatment and were associated with less major bleeding complications.
- In the extended treatment of venous thromboembolism, they showed superior efficacy compared with placebo. Clinically relevant bleeding was increased; however, the number of major bleeding was small.
- The benefit of the direct oral anticoagulants was confirmed also in special subgroups (eg, fragile patients) and in preliminary data from real-life clinical practice.

INTRODUCTION

Venous thromboembolism (VTE), including deep vein thrombosis (DVT) and pulmonary embolism (PE), is the third most common cardiovascular disease, after acute coronary syndromes and stroke.[1] The estimated incidence of VTE is 1 to 2 per 1000 person-years, with DVT accounting for two-thirds and PE accounting for the remaining one-third of the episodes.[2] VTE is a potentially fatal disorder, with an in-hospital case fatality rate associated with PE of approximately 10%, and it also carries a substantial

Dr N. Riva has no relevant conflicts to declare in relation to this article. Dr W. Ageno has participated in advisory boards for Bayer HealthCare, Boehringer Ingelheim, Bristol-Myers Squibb-Pfizer, and Daiichi Sankyo and has received travel or research support from Bayer HealthCare, GlaxoSmithKline, Pfizer-BMS, Daiichi-Sankyo, and Boehringer Ingelheim.
Department of Clinical and Experimental Medicine, University of Insubria, Via Guicciardini 9, Varese 21100, Italy
* Corresponding author.
E-mail addresses: agewal@yahoo.com; walter.ageno@uninsubria.it

Hematol Oncol Clin N Am 30 (2016) 1035–1051
http://dx.doi.org/10.1016/j.hoc.2016.05.008
0889-8588/16/$ – see front matter © 2016 Elsevier Inc. All rights reserved.

risk of short- and long-term recurrent events as well as morbidities such as the post-thrombotic syndrome and postembolic pulmonary hypertension.[3,4]

For many years, the standard of treatment for the large majority of VTE patients has been based on the use of heparins, either unfractionated heparin (UFH) or low-molecular-weight heparin (LMWH) followed by the oral vitamin K antagonists (VKA).[5] However, all these compounds had some limitations, including parenteral administration for heparins and the need for routine coagulation monitoring and dose adjustments for VKAs.[6] The direct oral anticoagulants (DOACs) have been developed to overcome some of these limitations.[7] The DOACs have a favorable pharmacologic profile (eg, fast onset and offset of action) and a predictable anticoagulant response, thus making their use particularly interesting for both the acute phase treatment and the long-term secondary prevention of VTE.

PHARMACOLOGIC PROPERTIES OF THE DIRECT ORAL ANTICOAGULANTS

The DOACs act on specific targets in the coagulation cascade. According to their specific target, they are classified as direct thrombin inhibitors (eg, dabigatran) and direct factor Xa inhibitors (eg, apixaban, rivaroxaban, and edoxaban).[6]

The onset of action ranges between 1 and 4 hours, thus allowing their use in the acute phase treatment of VTE, and the half-life ranges between 9 and 14 hours, thus allowing for a sufficiently rapid disappearance of the anticoagulant effect after discontinuation.[6] When compared with the VKAs, the DOACs have also a lower potential for food and drug interactions and a lower interindividual and intraindividual variability in dose response; thus, routine coagulation monitoring is not needed. The pharmacologic characteristics of the DOACs are summarized in **Table 1**.

Table 1
Pharmacologic properties of the direct oral anticoagulants

	Dabigatran	Rivaroxaban	Apixaban	Edoxaban
Mechanism of action	Direct thrombin inhibitor	Direct factor Xa inhibitor	Direct factor Xa inhibitor	Direct factor Xa inhibitor
Administration	Oral BID	Oral OD	Oral BID	Oral OD
Oral bioavailability	~ 6.5%	66% (without food) >80% (with food)	50%	62%
Time to peak plasma concentration	0.5–2 h	2–4 h	1–3 h	1–2 h
Mean half-life	12–14 h	5–9 h (young adult) 11–13 h (elderly)	~12 h	10–14 h
Renal clearance	85%	66% (only half as inactive metabolite)	27%	35%
Plasma protein binding	35% (dialyzable)	~90%	87%	~ 55%
Cytochrome P450 metabolism	No	Yes	Yes	Minimal
P-gp transport	Yes	Yes	Yes	Yes

Dabigatran binds to the active site of the thrombin molecule, therefore inactivating both free and fibrin-bound thrombin; in contrast, the indirect inhibitors of thrombin and factor Xa (such as UFH or LMWH) do not inactivate fibrin-bound thrombin, which can continue to stimulate thrombus expansion.[8] Dabigatran is orally administered as a prodrug, dabigatran etexilate. This formulation contains pellets of tartaric acid core coated with dabigatran etexilate and aims to create an acidic environment in the gastrointestinal tract, in order to reduce the variability in the absorption of the drug.[9] Dabigatran etexilate is hydrolyzed into the active form, dabigatran, by nonspecific esterase in the gut, plasma, and liver. Steady state is achieved after 3 days of multiple-dose administration in healthy volunteers.[10] Dabigatran has a low percentage of plasma protein binding of about 35%; therefore, it can be removed through dialysis. Approximately 80% is excreted unchanged through the kidney, while the remaining 20% is conjugated with glucuronic acid and excreted through the biliary system.[9] Dabigatran is not metabolized by the cytochrome P450 enzymes and is a substrate of the efflux transporter P-glycoprotein (P-gp), located in the intestine and kidneys. Therefore, potent inhibitors (eg, quinidine, ketoconazole, amiodarone, and verapamil) can increase dabigatran absorption and potent inducers (eg, rifampicin) can decrease dabigatran absorption.[8,11]

Rivaroxaban, apixaban, and edoxaban are direct inhibitors of the activated factor X (FXa), whereas the indirect inhibitors of thrombin and factor Xa require the cofactor antithrombin in order to inhibit factor Xa. They can bind directly not only free FXa but also FXa within the prothrombinase complex.[12–14]

The bioavailability of rivaroxaban after oral administration is dose-dependent: 80% to 100% is reported for the 10-mg dose and 66% for the 20-mg dose in the fasted state.[14] The administration with food results in delayed absorption but increased peak concentrations and is therefore recommended for therapeutic dosages.[15] One-third of the drug is excreted unchanged through the urine, while the other two-thirds are transformed into inactive metabolites and eliminated half by the renal route and half by the fecal route.[14] Rivaroxaban is a substrate for both cytochrome P450 enzymes and for P-gp transporter.

The bioavailability of apixaban is approximately 50% after oral administration,[16] and plasma protein binding in humans is 87%.[12] Several pathways are involved in the elimination of apixaban, each accounting for approximately one-third of the drug: hepatic metabolism, biliary and intestinal secretion, and renal clearance. Apixaban is a substrate of both cytochrome P450 and P-gp. However, apixaban has multiple elimination pathways, which can reduce the extent of drug-drug interaction. Conversely, apixaban does not significantly modulate the function of cytochrome P450 enzymes or P-gp transporter.[12,17]

Bioavailability of edoxaban after oral administration is 62%.[18] Edoxaban is transformed into several metabolites, mainly through hydrolysis; however, more than 70% is excreted unchanged. Approximately 35% of edoxaban is eliminated in the urine and 60% in the feces.[18,19] Edoxaban is a substrate of the P-gp transporter, while only a very small percentage (approximately 4%) is metabolized by cytochrome P450.

Being substrates of P-gp transporter and cytochrome P450 3A4, factor Xa inhibitors share common drug-drug interactions. Strong P-gp and CYP3A4 inhibitors, such as azole-antimycotics (ketoconazole, itraconazole, posaconazole, voriconazole) and HIV protease inhibitors (ritonavir), may increase their plasma concentration, whereas potent P-gp inducers, such as some antiepileptic drugs (carbamazepine, phenytoin, phenobarbital) and some antibiotics (rifampicin), may reduce their plasma concentration.

TREATMENT OF ACUTE VENOUS THROMBOEMBOLISM

Several randomized controlled trials investigated the use of the DOACs in patients with VTE. In the acute phase of treatment, dabigatran and edoxaban were administered after an initial course of parenteral anticoagulation, while rivaroxaban and apixaban were directly started as single drugs, using loading doses for the first few weeks.

Dabigatran was evaluated in the RE-COVER I and II trials, 2 randomized, double-blind and double-dummy trials in which more than 5000 patients with acute VTE, initially treated with parenteral anticoagulation (UFH or LMWH) for a median of 9 days, were randomized to fixed-dose dabigatran 150 mg twice daily (BID) or warfarin dose-adjusted to maintain an international normalized ratio (INR) between 2.0 and 3.0.[20,21] In both trials, dabigatran was noninferior to warfarin in the primary efficacy outcome of recurrent symptomatic VTE or VTE-related death, which occurred in 2.4% of patients treated with dabigatran versus 2.1% of patients treated with warfarin in RE-COVER I (hazard ratio [HR] 1.10, 95% confidence interval [CI] 0.65–1.84)[20] and in 2.3% versus 2.2%, respectively, in RE-COVER II (HR 1.08, 95% CI 0.64–1.80).[21] When the results of the 2 trials were pooled, the incidence of major bleeding and of major or clinically relevant nonmajor bleeding during the double-dummy period was significantly lower with dabigatran (1.0% vs 1.6%; HR 0.60, 95% CI 0.36–0.99, and 4.4% vs 7.7%; HR 0.56, 95% CI 0.45–0.71, respectively).[21] Dyspepsia was the only relevant side effect that emerged from these trials, reported in 1.0% to 2.9% of patients receiving dabigatran.

Rivaroxaban was evaluated in 2 open-label randomized controlled trials. The EINSTEIN-DVT trial enrolled 3449 patients with acute DVT,[22] whereas the EINSTEIN-PE trial enrolled 4833 patients with acute symptomatic PE, regardless of the concomitant presence of DVT.[23] In both trials, rivaroxaban was administered at a dosage of 15 mg BID for 21 days, followed by 20 mg once daily (OD) for 3, 6, or 12 months, and was compared with enoxaparin followed by VKAs. Rivaroxaban was noninferior to VKA with regard to the primary efficacy outcome of recurrent fatal or nonfatal VTE, which occurred in 2.1% patients on rivaroxaban and 3.0% patients on VKA in the EINSTEIN-DVT trial (HR 0.68, 95% CI 0.44–1.04)[22] and in 2.1% and 1.8%, respectively, in the EINSTEIN-PE trial (HR 1.12, 95% CI 0.75–1.68).[23] The principal safety outcome, a composite of major and clinically relevant bleeding, was similar in the 2 groups, occurring in 8.1% patients on rivaroxaban and 8.1% patients on VKA in the EINSTEIN-DVT trial (HR 0.97, 95% CI 0.76–1.22)[22] and in 10.3% and 11.4%, respectively, in the EINSTEIN-PE trial (HR 0.90, 95% CI 0.76–1.07).[23] However, in the EINSTEIN-PE trial, major bleeding complications were significantly less common with rivaroxaban (1.1% vs 2.2%; HR 0.49, 95% CI 0.31–0.79),[23] and this was also observed in a pooled analysis of the 2 EINSTEIN trials (1.0% vs 1.7%; HR 0.54, 95% CI 0.37–0.79).[24] Furthermore, in a post-hoc analysis of the EINSTEIN program, rivaroxaban was also associated with shorter hospital stay than enoxaparin/VKA (mean length of stay 4.5 vs 6.1 days).[25]

Apixaban was evaluated in the AMPLIFY trial, a double-blind double-dummy trial in which 5400 patients with acute VTE were randomized to apixaban 10 mg BID for 7 days, followed by 5 mg BID, or subcutaneous enoxaparin followed by warfarin (INR target range 2.0–3.0), for a total duration of 6 months.[26] Apixaban showed similar efficacy compared with warfarin, and the primary outcome of recurrent symptomatic VTE and VTE-related death occurred in 2.3% and 2.7%, respectively (relative risk [RR] 0.84, 95% CI 0.60–1.18). In addition, apixaban was associated with significantly less hemorrhagic complications, both major (0.6% vs 1.8%; RR 0.31, 95% CI 0.17–0.55) and major or clinically relevant nonmajor bleeding (4.3% vs 9.7%; RR 0.44, 95% CI 0.36–0.55).[26]

Edoxaban was evaluated in the Hokusai-VTE trial, a double-blind double-dummy trial in which 8292 patients with acute VTE, initially treated with enoxaparin or UFH, were randomized to edoxaban 60 mg OD or warfarin, dose adjusted in order to maintain the target INR 2.0 to 3.0.[27] The dose of edoxaban was reduced to 30 mg OD in the case of creatinine clearance 30 to 50 mL/min, body weight less than 60 kg, or concomitant treatment with potent P-gp inhibitors. The primary efficacy outcome was recurrent VTE or VTE-related death, and it was evaluated at the end of the whole 12-month study period, regardless of treatment duration. Edoxaban was noninferior to warfarin in the primary efficacy outcome, which occurred in 3.2% versus 3.5% (HR 0.98, 95% CI 0.70–1.13). The respective rates during the on-treatment period were 1.6% versus 1.9% (HR 0.82, 95% CI 0.60–1.14). Edoxaban showed a trend toward less major bleeding complications (1.4% vs 1.6%; HR 0.84, 95% CI 0.59–1.21) and was associated with lower rates of the composite safety outcome of major or clinically relevant bleeding (8.5% vs 10.3%; HR 0.81, 95% CI 0.71–0.94).

The results of the pivotal randomized controlled trials for the treatment of acute VTE with the DOACs are summarized in **Fig. 1**.

Several systematic reviews and meta-analyses pooled the results of these randomized controlled trials.[28,29] Compared with the standard regimen (LMWH followed by VKA), the DOACs were confirmed to be noninferior in terms of efficacy and showed a more favorable safety profile. The RR of major bleeding with the DOACs was approximately two-thirds of heparin/VKA, while the risk of fatal and intracranial bleeding was approximately one-third.[28,29] Although a trend toward more gastrointestinal bleeding with the DOACs was observed in trials conducted in patients with atrial fibrillation, the rate of major gastrointestinal bleeding did not appear to be increased in patients with acute VTE. Indeed, the overall number of gastrointestinal bleeding in VTE trials was smaller, and the baseline characteristics of the population were different (eg, younger age and lower prevalence of concomitant antiplatelet therapy).[29,30] Finally, the rate of clinically relevant nonmajor bleeding was also slightly reduced with the DOACs.

EXTENDED TREATMENT OF VENOUS THROMBOEMBOLISM

Several randomized controlled trials evaluated the DOACs for the extended treatment of VTE. Most of them compared the DOACs with placebo and aimed to demonstrate the superior efficacy of the active treatment in patients with clinical equipoise regarding the maintenance or discontinuation of the anticoagulant treatment. Only one compared a DOAC, dabigatran, with warfarin.

In the RE-MEDY trial, 2866 patients who had completed at least 3 months of anticoagulant treatment were randomized to dabigatran 150 mg BID or warfarin (INR target range 2.0–3.0).[31] The incidence of the primary endpoint of recurrent or fatal VTE was similar in the 2 groups (1.8% vs 1.3%, respectively; HR 1.44, 95% CI 0.78–2.64). Dabigatran showed a tendency toward a safer profile, with regards to major bleeding (0.9% vs 1.8%; HR 0.52, 95% CI 0.27–1.02) and the composite outcome of major or clinically relevant bleeding (5.6% vs 10.2%; HR 0.54, 95% CI 0.41–0.71).[31] However, more acute coronary syndromes were reported with the use of dabigatran (0.9% vs 0.2%), a finding that emerged also in studies evaluating patients with atrial fibrillation.[32] In the RE-SONATE trial, 1353 patients were randomized to dabigatran or placebo. Dabigatran met the criterion for superior efficacy in the primary outcome, a composite of recurrent or fatal VTE or unexplained death, which occurred in 0.4% and 5.6% of patients, respectively (HR 0.08, 95% CI 0.02–0.25, P<.001).[31] As expected, major or clinically relevant bleeding was higher with dabigatran (5.3% vs

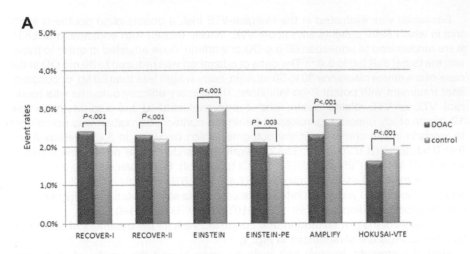

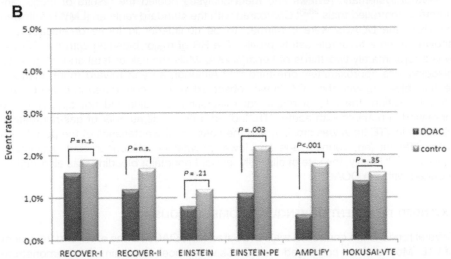

Fig. 1. Results of randomized controlled trials evaluating the DOACs for the acute treatment of VTE. (*A*) Efficacy: recurrent VTE or VTE-related death. These *P* values are for noninferiority. (*B*) Safety: major bleeding.

1.8%; HR 2.92, 95% CI 1.52–5.60), although the actual number of major bleeding events was small (2 vs 0 patients, respectively).

The EINSTEIN-Extension trial evaluated rivaroxaban 20 mg OD compared with placebo in 1197 patients who had completed 6 to 12 months of acute treatment of VTE.[22] Rivaroxaban was superior to placebo in the primary outcome of recurrent fatal or nonfatal VTE (1.3% vs 7.1%; HR 0.18, 95% CI 0.09–0.39). Major or clinically relevant bleeding occurred in 6.0% versus 1.2%, respectively (HR 5.19, 95% CI 2.3–11.7), whereas major bleeding occurred in 4 patients receiving rivaroxaban (0.7%) and 0 patients receiving placebo. Most of the clinically relevant nonmajor bleeding events were from mucosal sites and did not requires permanent discontinuation of anticoagulant treatment.[22] A lower dose of rivaroxaban (10 mg OD) for the extended treatment of VTE is currently being evaluated in the EINSTEIN-CHOICE trial, in comparison with the approved dose of rivaroxaban (20 mg OD) and with aspirin 100 mg daily.[33]

The AMPLIFY-EXT trial evaluated 2 doses of apixaban (2.5 mg and 5 mg BID) compared with placebo in 2486 patients who had completed 6 to 12 months of anti-coagulant treatment.[34] In this trial, the primary efficacy outcome was a composite of recurrent VTE and all-cause mortality and was significantly reduced with both dosages of apixaban (3.8% vs 11.6% for apixaban 2.5 mg BID and placebo, respectively, RR 0.33, 95% CI 0.22–0.48; and 4.2% vs 11.6% for apixaban 5 mg BID and placebo, respectively, RR 0.36, 95% CI 0.25–0.53). Furthermore, apixaban also reduced the rate of recurrent VTE or VTE-related death (1.7% vs 8.8% for apixaban 2.5 mg BID and placebo, respectively, RR 0.19, 95% CI 0.11–0.33; and 1.7% vs 8.8% for apixa-ban 5 mg BID and placebo, RR 0.20, 95% CI 0.11–0.34). No difference in efficacy emerged between the 2 apixaban dosages. The rate of major bleeding was not increased with apixaban (0.2% vs 0.5% for apixaban 2.5 mg BID and placebo, respec-tively, RR 0.49, 95% CI 0.09–2.64; and 0.1% vs 0.5% for apixaban 5 mg BID and pla-cebo, respectively, RR 0.25, 95% CI 0.03–2.24). Conversely, the composite safety outcome of major or clinically relevant bleeding showed a trend toward increased hemorrhagic risk with the higher dose of apixaban (2.7% in the placebo group, 3.2% in the apixaban 2.5 mg BID, and 4.3% in the apixaban 5 mg BID; RR 1.20, 95% CI 0.69–2.10, for the comparison apixaban 2.5 mg BID vs placebo; RR 1.62, 95% CI 0.96–2.73, for the comparison apixaban 5 mg BID vs placebo; and RR 0.74, 95% CI 0.46–1.22, for the comparison apixaban 2.5 mg BID vs 5 mg BID).

The results of the pivotal randomized controlled trials for the extended treatment of VTE with the DOACs compared with placebo are summarized in **Fig. 2**. When the re-sults of these 3 randomized controlled trials were pooled, recurrent VTE or VTE-related death occurred in 1.3% of patients receiving DOACs versus 7.3% of patients receiving placebo (odds ratio [OR] 0.16, 95% CI 0.11–0.24; number needed to treat 17), whereas major bleeding events occurred in 0.3% and 0.2%, respectively (OR 1.87, 95% CI 0.19–17.96). However, the rate of major or clinically relevant bleeding was significantly increased with the DOACs (4.6% vs 2.0%; OR 2.69, 95% CI 1.25–5.77; number needed to harm 39).[35]

TREATMENT OF SPECIAL POPULATIONS

Treatment of VTE might be particularly challenging in certain populations with a partic-ularly high risk of both bleeding complications and recurrent thrombotic events, such as the elderly, patients with renal impairment, or patients with cancer.[36]

A pooled analysis of the EINSTEIN trials focused on "fragile" patients (defined as age >75 years, creatinine clearance <50 mL/min, or body weight ≤50 kg), who repre-sented almost 20% of the population.[24] The overall rate of recurrent VTE and major bleeding was higher in fragile patients compared with nonfragile patients (3.2% vs 1.9% for recurrent VTE; 2.9% vs 1.0% for major bleeding). The use of rivaroxaban was associated with a significant reduction of major bleeding complications in fragile patients compared with the standard treatment (1.3% vs 4.5%, respectively; HR 0.27, 95% CI 0.13–0.54).[24] Similarly, in the Hokusai trial approximately 18% of the popula-tion qualified for the reduced dosage of edoxaban, because of creatinine clearance 30 to 50 mL/min, body weight ≤60 kg, or concomitant treatment with strong P-gp inhib-itors.[27] In these patients, edoxaban was associated with a significant reduction of clin-ically relevant bleeding compared with the standard treatment (7.9% vs 12.8%, respectively; HR 0.62, 95% CI 0.44–0.86).[27]

Anticoagulant treatment in oncologic patients is particularly difficult, due to several drug-drug interactions, as well as the frequent need for interruptions, like in case of bleeding, chemotherapy-induced thrombocytopenia, or invasive procedures.[36] So

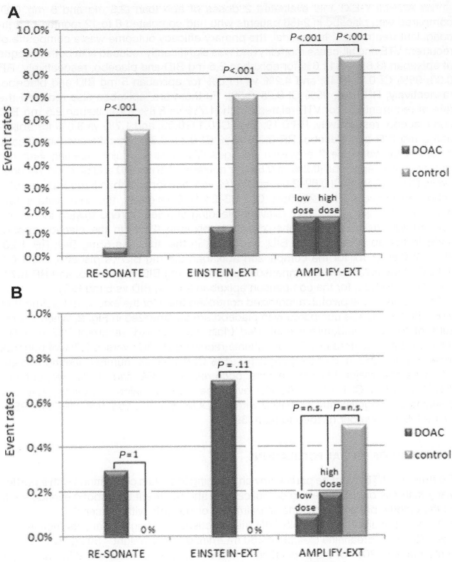

Fig. 2. Results of randomized controlled trials evaluating the DOACs for the extended treatment of VTE. (*A*) Efficacy: recurrent VTE or VTE-related death. (*B*) Safety: major bleeding.

far, there is preliminary evidence from subgroup analysis and meta-analysis of the randomized controlled trials that the efficacy and safety of the DOACs might be consistent also in these patients. A pooled analysis of the RECOVER-I and -II trials did not show any difference in the efficacy or safety of dabigatran among patients with cancer: the rate of recurrent VTE was 5.2% in patients receiving dabigatran and 7.4% in those receiving warfarin, whereas major bleeding occurred in 3.8% and 4.6%, respectively, without any significant treatment interaction by cancer status for both outcomes.[37] Overall, cancer was associated with a 3-fold higher risk of recurrence and 4-fold higher risk of major bleeding complications, compared with patients without cancer.[37]

In a pooled analysis of the EINSTEIN-DVT and PE studies, recurrent VTE occurred in 5.1% of patients with active cancer treated with rivaroxaban and 7.1% of patients treated with VKAs, and major bleeding occurred in 2.8% and 5.0%, respectively.[24] Similar results emerged from a subgroup analysis of patients with active cancer included in the AMPLIFY trial: the rate of recurrent VTE was 3.7% in patients receiving apixaban and 6.4% in patients receiving warfarin, while the corresponding rates of major bleeding were 2.3% and 5.0%.[38]

However, it should be noted that only approximately 5% of the patients enrolled in the randomized controlled trials had active cancer, that patients with more extensive disease were likely excluded, and that the DOACs were compared with VKAs and not to LMWH, the current standard of care for patients with cancer. An open-label randomized controlled trial specifically evaluating oncologic patients has been planned. The Hokusai-VTE Cancer study will enroll approximately 1000 patients with cancer with symptomatic or incidental PE or DVT and will compare edoxaban, administered at the same dose regimen of the Hokusai trial, with dalteparin 200 U/kg for 30 days, followed by 150 U/kg, for at least 6 months.[39] Considering the complexity of oncologic patients, the investigators established as primary outcome a composite of recurrent VTE and major bleeding.[39]

Only patients with hemodynamically stable PE were eligible for inclusion in the randomized controlled trials evaluating the DOACs in the acute phase treatment of VTE. Furthermore, it is likely that only a few patients with intermediate to high-risk PE were included in these studies. However, a subgroup analysis from the Hokusai trial provided data on patients with PE and right ventricular dysfunction as a measure of PE severity (defined as NT-proBNP $\geq$500 pg/mL), which represented almost one-third of the PE population. In this group, edoxaban was associated with a lower incidence of recurrent VTE compared with warfarin (3.3% vs 6.2%, respectively; HR 0.52, 95% CI 0.28–0.98).[27]

Asian patients have a higher risk of bleeding, and some guidelines recommend a reduced therapeutic intensity. For example, Japanese guidelines recommended warfarin to be administered at a lower INR range, between 1.5 and 2.5.[40] For this reason, specific randomized controlled trials or subgroups analysis was conducted in this population. The J-EINSTEIN DVT and PE program enrolled 100 patients with acute DVT or PE: 81 were randomized to rivaroxaban (10 mg or 15 mg BID for DVT patients and 15 mg BID for PE patients in the initial 3 weeks, followed by 15 mg OD) and 19 were randomized to the standard therapy (UFH followed by warfarin with INR target range 1.5–2.5).[41] The primary outcome consisted of a composite of symptomatic recurrent VTE and asymptomatic deterioration, which occurred in 1.4% patients receiving rivaroxaban versus 5.3% patients receiving standard treatment. There were no major bleeding complications in either group, whereas clinically relevant nonmajor bleeding occurred in 7.8% and 5.3%, respectively.[41] Therefore, the results of this study were consistent with the global EINSTEIN program. The AMPLIFY-J study randomized 80 Japanese subjects with acute DVT or PE to apixaban (10 mg BID for 7 days, followed by 5 mg BID up to 6 months) or UFH followed by warfarin.[42] Results were consistent with those of the AMPLIFY trial: apixaban showed similar efficacy than the standard treatment (0 vs 1 patient with recurrent VTE, respectively) and a trend toward less major or clinically relevant nonmajor bleeding (7.5% vs 28.2%).[42] Finally, a subgroup analysis of the Hokusai-VTE trial was specifically conducted in Asian patients.[43] Edoxaban was noninferior to warfarin in the primary outcome of recurrent VTE while on treatment (2.0% vs 2.0%; HR 0.96, 95% CI 0.42–2.20), and it was associated with lower rates of major or clinically relevant nonmajor bleeding complications (9.9% vs 17.3%; HR 0.56, 95% CI 0.40–0.78).[43]

Table 2
Dosage of the direct oral anticoagulant for the treatment of venous thromboembolism

	Dosage Studied in Phase III RCTs	Dosage Approved by the FDA	Dosage Approved by the EMA
Dabigatran	• Treatment of acute VTE: 150 mg BID, after initial parenteral anticoagulation for at least 5 d • Extended treatment of VTE: 150 mg BID	• Treatment of VTE: 150 mg BID, after 5–10 d of parenteral anticoagulation • Prevention of recurrent VTE: 150 mg BID • Avoid concomitant P-gp inducers (eg, rifampin) • Avoid concomitant P-gp inhibitors (eg, dronedarone, ketoconazole) if creatinine clearance <50 mL/min • No dosing recommendations if creatinine clearance ≤30 mL/min	• Treatment of VTE and prevention of recurrent VTE: 150 mg BID, following treatment with a parenteral anticoagulant for at least 5 d • Dose reduction to 110 mg BID if age ≥80 y or concomitant verapamil • Consider 150 mg BID or 110 mg BID based on individual assessment of thrombotic and bleeding risk in patients with age 75–80 y, moderate renal impairment, gastrointestinal diseases (gastritis, esophagitis, gastroesophageal reflux), or increased bleeding risk • Avoid concomitant P-gp inducers (eg, St. John's wort, carbamazepine, phenytoin) • Avoid concomitant strong P-gp inhibitors (eg, ketoconazole, cyclosporine, itraconazole, dronedarone) • Contraindicated in severe renal impairment (creatinine clearance <30 mL/min)
Rivaroxaban	• Treatment of acute VTE: 15 mg BID for 21 d, then 20 mg OD • Extended treatment of VTE: 20 mg OD	• Treatment of VTE: 15 mg BID for 21 d, then 20 mg OD • Prevention of recurrent VTE: 20 mg OD • Avoid rivaroxaban if creatinine clearance ≤30 mL/min • Avoid concomitant combined P-gp and strong CYP3A4 inhibitors (eg, ketoconazole, itraconazole, lopinavir, ritonavir, indinavir, and conivaptan) and inducers (eg, carbamazepine, phenytoin, rifampin, St. John's wort)	• Treatment of VTE: 15 mg BID for 21 d, then 20 mg OD • Prevention of recurrent VTE: 20 mg OD • Use with caution if creatinine clearance <30 mL/min. Not recommended if creatinine clearance <15 mL/min • In moderate-severe renal impairment (creatinine clearance 15–49 mL/min); after the initial 3 wk of treatment, a dose reduction to 15 mg OD can be considered if the bleeding risk outweighs the risk of recurrent VTE • Avoid concomitant combined P-gp and strong CYP3A4 inhibitors (eg, ketoconazole, itraconazole, voriconazole, posaconazole, ritonavir) and inducers (eg, rifampicin, phenytoin, carbamazepine, phenobarbital, St. John's wort)

Apixaban	• Treatment of acute VTE: 10 mg BID for 7 d, then 5 mg BID • Extended treatment of VTE: 2.5 mg BID or 5 mg BID	• Treatment of VTE: 10 mg BID for 7 d, followed by 5 mg BID • Prevention of recurrent VTE: 2.5 mg BID after at least 6 mo of treatment • No dose adjustment in renal impairment; however, no available data for patients with creatinine clearance <15 mL/min • Dose reduction by 50% if patients receiving 10 or 5 mg BID and concomitant strong dual inhibitors of CYP3A4 and P-gp (eg, ketoconazole, itraconazole, ritonavir, clarithromycin). Avoid these drugs if already taking 2.5 mg BID • Avoid concomitant strong dual inducers of CYP3A4 and P-gp (eg, rifampin, carbamazepine, phenytoin, St. John's wort)	• Treatment of VTE: 10 mg BID for 7 d, followed by 5 mg BID • Prevention of recurrent VTE: 2.5 mg BID after at least 6 mo of treatment • Use with caution if creatinine clearance <30 mL/min. Not recommended if creatinine clearance <15 mL/min • Avoid concomitant strong inhibitors of both CYP3A4 and P-gp (eg, ketoconazole, itraconazole, voriconazole, posaconazole, ritonavir) • Avoid concomitant strong inducers of both CYP3A4 and P-gp (eg, rifampicin, phenytoin, carbamazepine, phenobarbital, St. John's wort) for the treatment of acute VTE; use with caution for the prevention of recurrent VTE
Edoxaban	Treatment of acute VTE: 60 mg OD, after initial parenteral anticoagulation for at least 5 d. Dose reduced to 30 mg OD if creatinine clearance 30–50 mL/min, body weight ≤60 kg, or concomitant potent P-gp inhibitors (eg, verapamil, quinidine)	• Treatment of VTE: 60 mg OD, after 5–10 d of parenteral anticoagulation. Dose reduced to 30 mg OD if creatinine clearance 15–50 mL/min, body weight ≤60 kg, or concomitant P-gp inhibitors • Not recommended in patients with creatinine clearance <15 mL/min • Avoid concomitant P-gp inducers (eg, rifampin)	• Treatment of VTE and prevention of recurrent VTE: 60 mg OD, following treatment with a parenteral anticoagulant for at least 5 d • Dose reduced to 30 mg OD if creatinine clearance 15–50 mL/min, body weight ≤60 kg, or concomitant P-gp inhibitors (eg, ciclosporin, dronedarone, erythromycin, ketoconazole) • Not recommended in patients with creatinine clearance <15 mL/min • Concomitant P-gp inducers should be used with caution (eg, rifampicin, phenytoin, carbamazepine, phenobarbital, St. John's wort)

Abbreviations: EMA, European Medicines Agency; FDA, US Food and Drug Administration; RCT, randomized controlled trial.

Finally, there is currently no evidence regarding the use of the DOACs in patients with severe thrombophilia or unusual site VTE, although ongoing trials are testing rivaroxaban in patients with antiphospholipid syndrome[44] or in patients with splanchnic vein thrombosis.

USE OF THE DIRECT ORAL ANTICOAGULANTS IN ROUTINE CLINICAL PRACTICE

The DOACs have been licensed for the treatment of VTE in North America[45–48] and in the European Union,[49–52] and the approved dosages are reported in **Table 2**. The DOACs have also been mentioned by the recent guidelines of the European Society of Cardiology as alternatives to the current standard of care for the treatment of acute PE.[53]

Real-life data, coming from registries, will provide additional information in less selected patient populations. So far, preliminary results from the Dresden registry confirm the favorable safety profile of the DOACs in a real-world setting.[54] Several German hospitals and private practices contributed to this large, multicenter, prospective registry. Between October 2011 and December 2013, 1775 patients received rivaroxaban (1200 for AF and 575 for VTE). The median age of VTE patients was 68 years, therefore representing a population approximately 1 decade older compared with that included in the randomized controlled trials. The overall rate of major bleeding was 3.4 per 100 patient-years (95% CI 2.6–4.4).[54] Overall, there were 66 major bleeding events according to the definition of the International Society of Thrombosis and Haemostasis (6.1% of all bleeding complications), but only 9 patients required reversal strategies (3 prothrombin complex concentrates, 3 fresh frozen plasma, and 3 both). Case-fatality rate of major bleeding was low (5.1% at 30 days and 6.3% at 90 days after bleeding) compared with the case-fatality rate exceeding 10% usually reported for VKAs.[55]

XALIA is a noninterventional observational study in which approximately 4800 patients with DVT have been treated with rivaroxaban or the standard treatment (initial UFH, LMWH, or fondaparinux, overlapped with and followed by VKAs) for at least 3 months.[56] Enrollment in the XALIA study has been completed, and the results will be presented soon.

RE-COVERY is a noninterventional observational study that will enroll 6000 to 8000 patients with DVT or PE and planned anticoagulation therapy for at least 3 months.[57] Those receiving dabigatran or VKAs will be followed up for 1 year. The recruitment started the end of 2015, and the results are expected in 2019.

PREFER in VTE is another observational registry, which aims to enroll more than 4000 patients with DVT or PE from 7 European countries.[58] In this study, information about patient quality of life and treatment satisfaction is also collected.

The GARFIELD-VTE registry is actively enrolling VTE patients, with a target sample of 10,000 patients and a long-term follow-up.[59] The results are expected in 2018.

SUMMARY OF EVIDENCE

The key messages regarding the use of the DOACs in the treatment of VTE can be summarized as follows:

- In the acute treatment of VTE, the DOACs showed noninferior efficacy compared with the standard treatment (UFH or LMWH overlapped and followed by a VKA). When pooled, the risk of major bleeding complications was approximately two-thirds and the risk of fatal or intracranial bleeding was approximately one-third of standard treatment. The reduction in the rate of major bleeding was particularly evident for apixaban in the AMPLIFY trial, followed by rivaroxaban and dabigatran in the pooled analysis of the EINSTEIN and RECOVER trials, respectively.

- In the extended treatment of VTE, the DOACs showed superior efficacy compared with placebo. Clinically relevant bleeding was increased by the active treatment; however, the number of major bleeding was relatively small. In particular, 2 different dosages of apixaban have been evaluated, and the lower dosage has been approved by regulatory agencies, therefore allowing the continued secondary prevention of VTE with a lower risk of major bleeding complications. Furthermore, dabigatran is the only DOAC that has been directly compared with warfarin for this indication, showing a favorable safety profile.
- The benefit of the DOACs was confirmed also in special subgroups (eg, in fragile patients, in PE with right ventricular dysfunction, and in Asian patients). Additional data from clinical trials are warranted, in particular, in patients with cancer.
- Finally, the DOACs have specific pharmacologic properties that should be taken into account when prescribing these drugs. The predictable anticoagulant response does not require routine coagulation monitoring, whereas the rapid onset of action and the short half-life may allow short interruptions in the case of surgery or interventional procedures. Dabigatran and edoxaban are initiated after an initial course of parenteral treatment, while rivaroxaban and apixaban can be started immediately with a single-drug approach, with loading doses administered for 1 (apixaban) to 3 (rivaroxaban) weeks. Furthermore, rivaroxaban and edoxaban are administered OD, whereas dabigatran and apixaban require BID dosage; however, patient adherence is crucial with both dose regimens. Factor Xa inhibitors have multiple elimination pathways, whereas dabigatran has the highest rate of renal clearance and therefore needs to be used with caution in frail elderly patients with renal impairment. Finally, caution should also be applied with some interfering drugs.

In conclusion, the availability of the DOACs represents a new era in the treatment of VTE, due to the favorable efficacy and safety profile, the ease of use, and the potential for shorter hospital stay, compared with standard treatment. Preliminary data from registries seem to confirm the benefit of the DOACs in real-life clinical practice; however, further studies are needed to evaluate the long-term safety of these drugs.

REFERENCES

1. Goldhaber SZ. Venous thromboembolism: epidemiology and magnitude of the problem. Best Pract Res Clin Haematol 2012;25(3):235–42.
2. Naess IA, Christiansen SC, Romundstad P, et al. Incidence and mortality of venous thrombosis: a population-based study. J Thromb Haemost 2007;5(4): 692–9.
3. Dentali F, Ageno W, Pomero F, et al. Time trends and case fatality rate of in-hospital treated pulmonary embolism during 11 years of observation in Northwestern Italy. Thromb Haemost 2015;115(2):399–405.
4. Goldhaber SZ, Bounameaux H. Pulmonary embolism and deep vein thrombosis. Lancet 2012;379(9828):1835–46.
5. Kearon C, Akl EA, Comerota AJ, et al, American College of Chest Physicians. Antithrombotic therapy for VTE disease: antithrombotic therapy and prevention of thrombosis, 9th ed: American College of Chest Physicians evidence-based clinical practice guidelines. Chest 2012;141(2 Suppl):e419S–4194S.
6. Ageno W, Gallus AS, Wittkowsky A, et al, American College of Chest Physicians. Oral anticoagulant therapy: antithrombotic therapy and prevention of thrombosis,

9th ed: American College of Chest Physicians evidence-based clinical practice guidelines. Chest 2012;141(2 Suppl):e44S–88S.

7. Barnes GD, Ageno W, Ansell J, et al. Subcommittee on the control of anticoagulation. recommendation on the nomenclature for oral anticoagulants: communication from the SSC of the ISTH. J Thromb Haemost 2015;13(6):1154–6.

8. Hankey GJ, Eikelboom JW. Dabigatran etexilate: a new oral thrombin inhibitor. Circulation 2011;123(13):1436–50.

9. Eisert WG, Hauel N, Stangier J, et al. Dabigatran: an oral novel potent reversible nonpeptide inhibitor of thrombin. Arterioscler Thromb Vasc Biol 2010;30(10): 1885–9.

10. Stangier J, Rathgen K, Stähle H, et al. The pharmacokinetics, pharmacodynamics and tolerability of dabigatran etexilate, a new oral direct thrombin inhibitor, in healthy male subjects. Br J Clin Pharmacol 2007;64(3):292–303.

11. Stangier J, Clemens A. Pharmacology, pharmacokinetics, and pharmacodynamics of dabigatran etexilate, an oral direct thrombin inhibitor. Clin Appl Thromb Hemost 2009;15(Suppl 1):9S–16S.

12. Wong PC, Pinto DJ, Zhang D. Preclinical discovery of apixaban, a direct and orally bioavailable factor Xa inhibitor. J Thromb Thrombolysis 2011;31(4):478–92.

13. Furugohri T, Isobe K, Honda Y, et al. DU-176b, a potent and orally active factor Xa inhibitor: in vitro and in vivo pharmacological profiles. J Thromb Haemost 2008; 6(9):1542–9.

14. Perzborn E, Roehrig S, Straub A, et al. Rivaroxaban: a new oral factor Xa inhibitor. Arterioscler Thromb Vasc Biol 2010;30(3):376–81.

15. Kubitza D, Becka M, Zuehlsdorf M, et al. Effect of food, an antacid, and the H2 antagonist ranitidine on the absorption of BAY 59-7939 (rivaroxaban), an oral, direct factor Xa inhibitor, in healthy subjects. J Clin Pharmacol 2006;46(5): 549–58.

16. Roser-Jones C, Becker RC. Apixaban: an emerging oral factor Xa inhibitor. J Thromb Thrombolysis 2010;29(1):141–6.

17. Raghavan N, Frost CE, Yu Z, et al. Apixaban metabolism and pharmacokinetics after oral administration to humans. Drug Metab Dispos 2009;37(1):74–81.

18. Lip GY, Agnelli G. Edoxaban: a focused review of its clinical pharmacology. Eur Heart J 2014;35(28):1844–55.

19. Bounameaux H, Camm AJ. Edoxaban: an update on the new oral direct factor xa inhibitor. Drugs 2014;74(11):1209–31.

20. Schulman S, Kearon C, Kakkar AK, et al, RE-COVER Study Group. Dabigatran versus warfarin in the treatment of acute venous thromboembolism. N Engl J Med 2009;361(24):2342–52.

21. Schulman S, Kakkar AK, Goldhaber SZ, et al, RE-COVER II Trial Investigators. Treatment of acute venous thromboembolism with dabigatran or warfarin and pooled analysis. Circulation 2014;129(7):764–72.

22. EINSTEIN Investigators, Bauersachs R, Berkowitz SD, et al. Oral rivaroxaban for symptomatic venous thromboembolism. N Engl J Med 2010;363(26):2499–510.

23. EINSTEIN–PE Investigators, Büller HR, Prins MH, et al. Oral rivaroxaban for the treatment of symptomatic pulmonary embolism. N Engl J Med 2012;366(14): 1287–97.

24. Prins MH, Lensing AW, Bauersachs R, et al, EINSTEIN Investigators. Oral rivaroxaban versus standard therapy for the treatment of symptomatic venous thromboembolism: a pooled analysis of the EINSTEIN-DVT and PE randomized studies. Thromb J 2013;11(1):21.

25. Bookhart BK, Haskell L, Bamber L, et al. Length of stay and economic consequences with rivaroxaban vs enoxaparin/vitamin K antagonist in patients with DVT and PE: findings from the North American EINSTEIN clinical trial program. J Med Econ 2014;17(10):691–5.

26. Agnelli G, Buller HR, Cohen A, et al, AMPLIFY Investigators. Oral apixaban for the treatment of acute venous thromboembolism. N Engl J Med 2013;369(9): 799–808.

27. Hokusai-VTE Investigators, Büller HR, Décousus H, et al. Edoxaban versus warfarin for the treatment of symptomatic venous thromboembolism. N Engl J Med 2013;369(15):1406–15.

28. van der Hulle T, Kooiman J, den Exter PL, et al. Effectiveness and safety of novel oral anticoagulants as compared with vitamin K antagonists in the treatment of acute symptomatic venous thromboembolism: a systematic review and meta-analysis. J Thromb Haemost 2014;12(3):320–8.

29. van Es N, Coppens M, Schulman S, et al. Direct oral anticoagulants compared with vitamin K antagonists for acute venous thromboembolism: evidence from phase 3 trials. Blood 2014;124(12):1968–75.

30. Caldeira D, Barra M, Ferreira A, et al. Systematic review with meta-analysis: the risk of major gastrointestinal bleeding with non-vitamin K antagonist oral anticoagulants. Aliment Pharmacol Ther 2015;42(11–12):1239–49.

31. Schulman S, Kearon C, Kakkar AK, et al, RE-MEDY Trial Investigators, RE-SONATE Trial Investigators. Extended use of dabigatran, warfarin, or placebo in venous thromboembolism. N Engl J Med 2013;368(8):709–18.

32. Uchino K, Hernandez AV. Dabigatran association with higher risk of acute coronary events: meta-analysis of noninferiority randomized controlled trials. Arch Intern Med 2012;172(5):397–402.

33. Weitz JI, Bauersachs R, Beyer-Westendorf J, et al, EINSTEIN CHOICE Investigators. Two doses of rivaroxaban versus aspirin for prevention of recurrent venous thromboembolism. Rationale for and design of the EINSTEIN CHOICE study. Thromb Haemost 2015;114(3):645–50.

34. Agnelli G, Buller HR, Cohen A, et al, AMPLIFY-EXT Investigators. Apixaban for extended treatment of venous thromboembolism. N Engl J Med 2013;368(8): 699–708.

35. Sardar P, Chatterjee S, Mukherjee D. Efficacy and safety of new oral anticoagulants for extended treatment of venous thromboembolism: systematic review and meta-analyses of randomized controlled trials. Drugs 2013;73(11):1171–82.

36. Prandoni P. Treatment of patients with acute deep vein thrombosis and/or pulmonary embolism: efficacy and safety of non-VKA oral anticoagulants in selected populations. Thromb Res 2014;134(2):227–33.

37. Schulman S, Goldhaber SZ, Kearon C, et al. Treatment with dabigatran or warfarin in patients with venous thromboembolism and cancer. Thromb Haemost 2015;114(1):150–7.

38. Agnelli G, Buller HR, Cohen A, et al. Oral apixaban for the treatment of venous thromboembolism in cancer patients: results from the AMPLIFY trial. J Thromb Haemost 2015;13(12):2187–91.

39. van Es N, Di Nisio M, Bleker SM, et al. Edoxaban for treatment of venous thromboembolism in patients with cancer. Rationale and design of the Hokusai VTE-cancer study. Thromb Haemost 2015;114(6):1268–76.

40. JCS Joint Working Group. Guidelines for the diagnosis, treatment and prevention of pulmonary thromboembolism and deep vein thrombosis (JCS 2009). Circ J 2011;75(5):1258–81.

41. Yamada N, Hirayama A, Maeda H, et al. Oral rivaroxaban for Japanese patients with symptomatic venous thromboembolism - the J-EINSTEIN DVT and PE program. Thromb J 2015;13:2.

42. Nakamura M, Nishikawa M, Komuro I, et al. Apixaban for the treatment of Japanese subjects with acute venous thromboembolism (AMPLIFY-J Study). Circ J 2015;79(6):1230–6.

43. Nakamura M, Wang YQ, Wang C, et al. Efficacy and safety of edoxaban for treatment of venous thromboembolism: a subanalysis of East Asian patients in the Hokusai-VTE trial. J Thromb Haemost 2015;13(9):1606–14.

44. Cohen H, Doré CJ, Clawson S, et al, RAPS Trial Protocol Collaborators. Rivaroxaban in antiphospholipid syndrome (RAPS) protocol: a prospective, randomized controlled phase II/III clinical trial of rivaroxaban versus warfarin in patients with thrombotic antiphospholipid syndrome, with or without SLE. Lupus 2015;24(10):1087–94.

45. Available at: http://wwwaccessdatafdagov/drugsatfda_docs/label/2015/022512s027lblpdf. Accessed October 24, 2015.

46. Food and Drug Administration. Eliquis (apixaban): highlights of prescribing information. Available at: http://wwwaccessdatafdagov/drugsatfda_docs/label/2015/202155s011lblpdf. Accessed October 24, 2015.

47. Food and Drug Administration. Xarelto (rivaroxaban): highlights of prescribing information. Available at: http://wwwaccessdatafdagov/drugsatfda_docs/label/2015/202439s015lblpdf. Accessed October 24, 2015.

48. Food and Drug Administration. Savaysa (edoxaban): highlights of prescribing information. Available at: http://wwwaccessdatafdagov/drugsatfda_docs/label/2015/206316s002lblpdf. Accessed October 24, 2015.

49. European Medicines Agency. Pradaxa (dabigatran etexilate): summary of product characteristics. Available at: http://wwwemaeuropaeu/docs/en_GB/document_library/EPAR_-_Product_Information/human/000829/WC500041059pdf. Accessed October 24, 2015.

50. European Medicines Agency. Eliquis (apixaban): summary of product characteristics. Available at: http://wwwemaeuropaeu/docs/en_GB/document_library/EPAR_-_Product_Information/human/002148/WC500107728pdf. Accessed October 24, 2015.

51. European Medicines Agency. Xarelto (rivaroxaban): summary of product characteristics. Available at: http://wwwemaeuropaeu/docs/en_GB/document_library/EPAR_-_Product_Information/human/000944/WC500057108pdf. Accessed October 24, 2015.

52. European Medicines Agency. Lixiana (edoxaban): summary of product characteristics. Available at: http://wwwemaeuropaeu/docs/en_GB/document_library/EPAR_-_Product_Information/human/002629/WC500189045pdf. Accessed October 24, 2015.

53. Konstantinides SV, Torbicki A, Agnelli G, et al. 2014 ESC guidelines on the diagnosis and management of acute pulmonary embolism. Eur Heart J 2014;35(43):3033–69, 3069a–k.

54. Beyer-Westendorf J, Förster K, Pannach S, et al. Rates, management, and outcome of rivaroxaban bleeding in daily care: results from the Dresden NOAC registry. Blood 2014;124(6):955–62.

55. Linkins LA, Choi PT, Douketis JD. Clinical impact of bleeding in patients taking oral anticoagulant therapy for venous thromboembolism: a meta-analysis. Ann Intern Med 2003;139(11):893–900.

56. Ageno W, Mantovani LG, Haas S, et al. XALIA: rationale and design of a non-interventional study of rivaroxaban compared with standard therapy for initial and long-term anticoagulation in deep vein thrombosis. Thromb J 2014;12:16.
57. Goldhaber SZ, Ageno W, Casella I, et al. A global prospective cohort study of dabigatran for the treatment of venous thromboembolism (RE-COVERY). J Thromb Haemost 2015;13(Suppl 2):729 [abstract: PO613-TUE].
58. Agnelli G, Gitt AK, Bauersachs R, et al, PREFER in VTE Investigators. The management of acute venous thromboembolism in clinical practice - study rationale and protocol of the European PREFER in VTE Registry. Thromb J 2015;13:41.
59. Beyer-Westendorf J, Ageno W. Benefit-risk profile of non-vitamin K antagonist oral anticoagulants in the management of venous thromboembolism. Thromb Haemost 2015;113(2):231–46.

Use of Direct Oral Anticoagulants in Special Populations

Ang Li, MD[a],*, Renato D. Lopes, MD, PhD[b], David A. Garcia, MD[c]

KEYWORDS

• DOAC • Anticoagulation • Venous thromboembolism • Atrial fibrillation

KEY POINTS

• Although direct oral anticoagulants (DOACs) represent an excellent alternative to warfarin in venous thrombosis or atrial fibrillation, some patient populations were not well-represented in individual clinical trials.

• For patients with extremes of body weight, advanced age, or moderate renal insufficiency, some DOACs may be preferred over warfarin and others may be less attractive.

• The choice and dosing of DOACs in selected populations is complex and must be individualized.

• More evidence about the safety and effectiveness of DOACs are needed in highly prothrombotic states, such as cancer and antiphospholipid syndrome.

INTRODUCTION

Although direct oral anticoagulants (DOACs) have been approved for the treatment of venous thromboembolism (VTE) and atrial fibrillation (AF) in the United States based on phase III randomized controlled trials (RCTs) that have directly compared with vitamin K antagonists (VKAs), questions remain about their applicability and safety in selected populations that were less represented in the trials. With rare exceptions, DOACs have been studied and approved using a "one-dose-fits-all" model, without

Conflict of Interest Disclosure: D.A. Garcia has served as a consultant to Boehringer Ingelheim, Bristol Meyers Squibb, Daiichi Sankyo, Janssen and Pfizer. R.D. Lopes has served as a consultant to Bayer, Boehringer Ingelheim, Bristol Myers Squibb, Glaxo Smith Kline, Merck, Pfizer and Portola.
[a] Division of Hematology, Department of Medicine, University of Washington Medical Center, University of Washington School of Medicine, 1959 NE Pacific St, Seattle, WA 98195, USA; [b] Division of Cardiology, Department of Medicine, Duke University Medical Center, Box 3850, 2400 Pratt Street, Room 0311, Terrace Level, Durham, NC 27705, USA; [c] Division of Hematology, Department of Medicine, University of Washington Medical Center, University of Washington School of Medicine, 1705 Northeast Pacific Street, Box 357710, Seattle, WA 98195, USA
* Corresponding author.
E-mail address: ali2015@uw.edu

the need for routine measurement of anticoagulant effect. Although this simplicity is attractive, in some situations, the absence of an evidence based dose adjustment algorithm can be problematic. In this article, we review the currently available evidence relevant to the use of DOACs in patients with extremes of body weight, advanced age, renal impairment, cancer, and antiphospholipid antibody syndrome (APS). When presenting data derived from individual or pooled subgroup analyses, both the interaction effects and the sample sizes within these subgroups are important. In **Table 1** we present the names of the major phase III VTE and AF trials, their relevant dosing, as well as the sample size for each subgroup. In this review, we will focus on the US Food and Drug Administration (FDA)–approved dosing when more than 1 dose has been studied for a particular DOAC.

PATIENTS AT EXTREMES OF BODY WEIGHT

Patients with extreme body weight are common in clinical practice. Obesity is an independent risk factor for both VTE and AF.[1–3] Alternatively, patients with low body weight may have higher risk of bleeding with all forms of anticoagulation. Pharmacokinetic and pharmacodynamic studies in healthy subjects suggest that overall DOAC exposure for patients at extremes of body weight (<50 or >120 kg) is not substantially different from the exposure in patients who weigh between 50 and 120 kg.[4–7] However, few patients with weight 50 kg or less or greater than 120 kg were included in phase III RCTs. While there is a metaanalysis comparing the efficacy and risks of DOACs versus VKA using data from the VTE (not AF) trials, the authors compared "clinically relevant" rather than "major bleeding" risks as a clinical outcome and there was significant variation of the definition of "high" and "low" body weight depending on the individual trial.[8] In this section, we review data from subgroups of phase III AF and VTE trials to compare the rates of thrombosis and major bleeding for DOACs versus VKA in patients with extremes of body weight (**Table 2**).

According to the package insert, dabigatran trough concentration is 20% lower in subjects with a body weight of greater than 100 kg.[4] In a pooled analysis of the Efficacy and Safety of Dabigatran Compared to Warfarin for 6 Month Treatment of Acute Symptomatic Venous Thromboembolism (RE-COVER) studies (see **Table 1**), dabigatran 150 mg versus warfarin had a consistent treatment effect on primary efficacy in both high (>100 kg) and low (≤50 kg) body weight subgroups (nonsignificant interactions).[9,10] Of note, there were only 57 patients with weight 50 kg or less and the number of patients with weight greater than 120 kg was not reported; thus, these results must be applied to these subgroups with caution. Major bleeding was not reported as a subgroup outcome. In the Randomized Evaluation of Long-term Anticoagulation Therapy (RE-LY) trial, subgroup analysis for dabigatran 150 mg versus warfarin based on weight was also consistent with the primary trial for both improved primary efficacy and noninferior major bleeding (nonsignificant interactions).[11,12] This result was confirmed by a recently published subgroup analysis where no significant interaction was observed for the relative effect of dabigatran versus warfarin on stroke or bleeding rates when patients were stratified into top 10% and bottom 10% of body mass index (BMI).[13]

When given to healthy volunteers, the area under the curve (AUC) for rivaroxaban was not significantly different ($P = .21$) for healthy subjects who weighed 50 kg or less or more than 120 kg when compared with those who weighed 70 to 80 kg.[5] In a pooled analysis of the 2 Oral Direct Factor Xa Inhibitor Rivaroxaban in Patients With Acute Symptomatic Deep Vein Thrombosis (EINSTEIN) VTE studies, there were only 107 patients with body weight of 50 kg or less.[14] In this low body weight

Table 1
Characteristics and number of patients included in specific subgroups for all major phase III clinical trials

Trial Name	Study	Year	Duration	Dosing	Total N	BW ≤60 kg	BW >100 kg	Age ≥75 y	eCrCl 30–50 mL/min	Cancer
Dabigatran										
RECOVER I/II[9,10]	VTE	2009/14	6 mo	150 bid	5107	57[d]	832	529	245	221
RE-LY[11]	AF	2009	24 mo	150/110 bid	18,113	376[d]	3099	7258[12]	3505	n.r.
Rivaroxaban										
EINSTEIN-DVT[15]	DVT	2010	3, 6, 12 mo	20 qd[h]	3449	86[d]	491	438	235	207
EINSTEIN-PE[16]	PE	2012	3, 6, 12 mo	20 qd[h]	4832	81[d]	704	843	398	223
ROCKET-AF[a,17]	AF	2011	23 mo	20 qd	14,262	4025[e]	3977[f]	6164	2949	n.r.
Apixaban										
AMPLIFY 2013[18]	VTE	2013	6 mo	5 bid[h]	5395	473	1039	768	338[i]	143
ARISTOTLE 2011[19]	AF	2011	22 mo	5 bid[b]	18,201	1985	7159[9,20]	5678	3017[i]	n.r.
Edoxaban										
HOKUSAI[23]	VTE	2013	3–12 mo	60 qd[c]	8240	1043	1265	1104	541	208[48]
ENGAGE-AF-TIMI[24]	AF	2013	34 mo	60/30 qd[c]	21,105	2083	n.r.	8474	4074	n.r.

Abbreviations: AF, atrial fibrillation; bid, twice daily; BW, body weight; DVT, deep vein thrombosis; eCrCl, estimated creatinine clearance calculated using the Cockcroft-Gault equation; n.r., not reported; PE, pulmonary embolism; qd, daily; VTE, venous thromboembolism.

a Data interpretation according to the intention to treat analysis.
b Lower dose if 2 of the following: Cr ≥1.5 mg/dL, age ≥80, or BW ≤60 kg.
c Lower dose if any of the following: eCrCl 30 to 50 mL/min, BW ≤60, or verapamil/quinidine/dronedarone (P-glycoprotein inhibitors).
d Variations in weight category depending on individual trial design (BW ≤50 kg).
e Variations in weight category depending on individual trial design (BW ≤70 kg).
f Variations in weight category depending on individual trial design (BW >90 kg).
g Variations in weight category depending on individual trial design (BMI >30).
h Dosing after initial loading dose.
i CrCl 25 to 50 mL/min.

Table 2
DOAC use in patients with extremes of body weight: relative effects versus VKA in phase III trials

	Primary Efficacy, DOAC vs VKA		Major Bleeding, DOAC vs VKA	
	BW ≤60 kg	BW >100 kg	BW ≤60 kg	BW >100 kg
Dabigatran 150 mg				
RECOVER I/II[10]	0 vs 3.2%/study (NS)[d]	4.1 vs 3.6%/study (NS)	n.r.	n.r.
RE-LY[11,12]	2.2 vs 5.0%/ly (NS)[d]	0.9 vs 0.9%/ly (NS)	4.9 vs 6.0%/ly (NS)[d]	4.0 vs 3.3%/y (NS)
Interpretation	Lower stroke/SE and noninferior recurrent VTE	Lower stroke/SE and noninferior recurrent VTE	Noninferior bleeding	Noninferior bleeding
Rivaroxaban 20 mg				
EINSTEIN-DVT/PE[14–16]	7.1 vs 3.0%/study (NS)[d]	2.0 vs 1.8%/study (NS)[f]	0 vs 4.6% (NS)[d]	n.r.
ROCKET-AF[a,17]	2.4 vs 2.8%/ly (NS)[e]	1.3 vs 1.2%/ly (NS)[f]	n.r.	n.r.
Interpretation	Noninferior recurrent VTE and stroke/SE	Noninferior recurrent VTE and stroke/SE	Insufficient data	Insufficient data
Apixaban 5 mg				
AMPLIFY[18]	2.7 vs 4.3%/study (NS)	2.2 vs 3.5%/study (NS)	0.4 vs 2.9%/study (NS)	0.2 vs 1.9%/study (sig)
ARISTOTLE[b,19,20]	2.0 vs 3.2%/ly (sig)	1.0 vs 1.3%/ly (NS)[g]	2.3 vs 4.3%/ly (sig)	2.1 vs 2.5%/y (NS)[g,h]
Interpretation	Lower stroke/SE and noninferior recurrent VTE	Lower stroke/SE[i] and Noninferior recurrent VTE	Lower bleeding for both VTE and AF	Lower bleeding for VTE, noninferior bleeding for AF
Edoxaban 60 mg				
HOKUSAI-VTE[c,23]	2.9 vs 3.5%/study (NS)	3.6 vs 3.5%/study (NS)	n.r.	n.r.
ENGAGE-TIMI-AF[c,24]	n.r.	n.r.	n.r.	n.r.
Interpretation	Noninferior recurrent VTE	Noninferior recurrent VTE	Insufficient data	Insufficient data

Abbreviations: AF, atrial fibrillation; BW, body weight; DOAC, direct oral anticoagulants; n.r., not reported; NS, nonsignificant; SE, systemic embolism; sig, significant; VKA, vitamin K antagonist; VTE, venous thromboembolism.

a Data interpretation according to the intention to treat analysis, percent per year is calculated by dividing reported event rate over median follow-up of study.

b Lower dose if 2 of the following: creatinine ≥1.5 mg/dL, age ≥80, or BW ≤60 kg.

c Lower dose if any of the following: estimated creatinine clearance using the Cockcroft-Gault equation of 30 to 50, BW ≤60, or verapamil/quinidine/dronedarone (P-glycoprotein inhibitors).

d Variations in weight category depending on individual trial design (BW ≤50 kg).

e Variations in weight category depending on individual trial design (BW ≤70 kg).

f Variations in weight category depending on individual trial design (BW ≤60 kg).

g Variations in weight category depending on individual trial design (BMI >90 kg).

h Variations in weight category depending on individual trial design (BMI >30).

i Significant interaction between treatment and BMI for indicated subgroup (interaction $P = .02$).

i Interpretation (lower stroke/SE) extrapolated from the primary trial as the interaction term was nonsignificant.

subgroup, there were not sufficient numbers to detect a difference in primary efficacy or major bleeding (nonsignificant interactions). Both EINSTEIN studies analyzed weight greater than 90 kg in the subgroups.[15,16] In this high body weight subgroup, there was no difference in primary efficacy (nonsignificant interactions) and major bleeding was not reported. In the Efficacy and safety of rivaroxaban compared with warfarin among elderly patients with nonvalvular atrial fibrillation in the rivaroxaban once daily, oral, direct factor Xa inhibition compared with vitamin K antagonism for prevention of stroke and embolism trial in atrial fibrillation (ROCKET-AF) trial, body weight subgroup used a different cutoff of 70 kg or less and greater than 90 kg.[17] There was no obvious difference in primary efficacy outcomes (nonsignificant interactions). Major bleeding was not reported in the weight-based subgroup analysis.

In pharmacokinetic studies of healthy volunteers, apixaban has a 20% higher AUC in subjects who weigh less than 50 kg and 23% lower AUC in those whose weight is greater than 120 kg compared with the reference group whose weight is 65 to 85 kg.[6] In the Apixaban for the Initial Management of Pulmonary Embolism and Deep-Vein Thrombosis as First-Line Therapy (AMPLIFY) trial, the subgroup analysis based on patients with high (>100 kg) or low (≤60 kg) body weight showed an effect consistent with the overall trial: no difference in recurrent VTE or death but significantly less major bleeding in the apixaban group in comparison with the VKA group (nonsignificant interactions).[18] In the Apixaban for Reduction in Stroke and Other Thromboembolic Events in Atrial Fibrillation (ARISTOTLE) trial, apixaban was dose-reduced for patients with weight 60 kg or less when another risk factor was present (creatinine ≥1.5 mg/dL or age ≥80 y). The subgroup analysis based on low body weight showed results consistent with the overall trial, which demonstrated both significantly decreased stroke/systemic embolism as well as significantly decreased major bleeding (nonsignificant interactions) for apixaban versus VKA.[19] In a recent subgroup analysis, 6.5% of the patients studied were found to have BMI >= 40. There was a significant interaction (interaction $P = .02$) between BMI categories and effects of apixaban versus warfarin concerning major bleeding, where apixaban use in patients with higher BMI (>30) was associated with less reduction in bleeding risk (hazard ratio [HR], 0.84; 0.67–1.07) when compared with patients with normal BMI (HR, 0.73, 0.57–0.92) or low BMI (HR, 0.51, 0.39–0.67).[20]

The pharmacokinetics of edoxaban dosing have been studied in several phase II dose-finding studies in patients with AF.[7] In a study of 536 Japanese AF patients, Yamashita and associates[21] found that minimum concentration of edoxaban was higher in those with weight less than 60 kg across all doses of the drug. In a study of 235 Asian AF patients, Chung and colleagues[22] confirmed that low body weight (≤60 kg) was associated with a higher minimum concentration of edoxaban and a higher incidence of bleeding. Consequently, subsequent phase III trials of edoxaban incorporated a "low-dose" edoxaban regimen (one-half dose of study drug) in patients with a weight of 60 kg or less. In the Evaluation of Efficacy and Safety of (LMW) Heparin/Edoxaban Versus (LMW) Heparin/Warfarin in Subjects With Symptomatic Deep-Vein Thrombosis and or Pulmonary Embolism (HOKUSAI-VTE) subgroup analysis with both high (>100 kg) and low (≤60 kg) body weights, edoxaban 60 mg had a consistent noninferior primary efficacy treatment effect compared with VKA (nonsignificant interactions).[23] Major bleeding was not reported in subgroups defined by weight. In the Global Study to Assess the Safety and Effectiveness of Edoxaban (DU-176b) vs Standard Practice of Dosing With Warfarin in Patients With Atrial Fibrillation (ENGAGE AF-TIMI 48) study, edoxaban 60 mg was noninferior to VKA for prevention of stroke/systemic embolism and had significantly lower rates of major bleeding.[24] Although there was further reduction in major bleeding in the dose-reduced groups (which included patients with low body weight), specific subgroup analysis on body weight was not reported.

In conclusion, there are sufficient data to show that, for major bleeding, apixaban 5 mg twice daily is superior to VKA in lower body weight subgroups (after necessary adjustment for age and estimated creatinine clearance [eCrCl]) and dabigatran 150 mg twice daily is noninferior to VKA in both high and low body weight subgroups. However, for the other 2 DOACs, more high-quality data are needed to exclude a possible effect of extreme body weight on the relative risk for major bleeding compared with VKA. DOACs (when used according to their labelling) seem to be non-inferior or superior to VKA for primary efficacy in both VTE and AF, even in patients weighing less than 50 kg or more than 100 kg. However, to the best of our knowledge, very few patients who weighed more than 120 kg were enrolled in the large phase III RCTs and there is likely a weight above which the anticoagulant effect of any DOAC would be insufficient.[25] Thus, more information about the efficacy and safety of FDA-approved doses of DOACs in extremely obese patients is needed.

ELDERLY PATIENTS OVER 75 YEARS OF AGE

Elderly patients pose another challenge because they have a heightened risk of both AF-related stroke and VTE.[26,27] Advanced age is also independently associated with a higher risk of major anticoagulation-associated bleeding, regardless of the type of anticoagulant used.[12,28] With the exception of apixaban for stroke prevention in AF treatment, phase III clinical trials of the DOACs did not specify dose reduction based on age. Several studies have analyzed the effect of DOACs by age, and a recent meta-analysis has pooled the combined bleeding risks of all DOACs.[29] Because different DOAC possess different bleeding risks in the elderly depending on the body site, available evidence is presented in this section with attention to overall major bleeding, intracranial bleeding, and gastrointestinal (GI) bleeding (**Table 3**).

For dabigatran, pharmacokinetic and pharmacodynamic study in healthy older subjects showed a statistically but not clinically significant increase in AUC; thus, dose adjustment for the elderly was not included in the registration trials.[30] A pooled subgroup analysis of the RE-COVER studies (see **Table 1**) showed no interaction between age and relative efficacy of dabigatran 150 mg versus VKA. The "major and clinically relevant" bleeding risk reduction was influenced by age (interaction $P = .01$): dabigatran 150 mg was associated with less bleeding in younger patients and more bleeding in those over age 85.[10] However, a dedicated analysis for major bleeding alone was not reported. In 7238 patients over age 75 from the RE-LY trial, dabigatran 150 mg was superior to VKA for the primary efficacy endpoint of stroke and systemic embolism (nonsignificant interaction for age on treatment effect). However, for bleeding risk, there was a significant treatment-by-age interaction ($P<.001$) whereby dabigatran 150 mg versus VKA was associated with a lower major bleeding risk in patients less than 75 years (RR, 0.70; 95% CI 0.57–0.86) and a trend toward higher major bleeding risk in patients 75 years and older (RR, 1.18; 95% CI 0.98–1.42).[12] Dabigatran 150 mg was associated with both decreased intracranial bleeding risk and increased major GI bleeding risk in all age groups, although the increased risk of GI bleeding seemed to be more pronounced in those over 75 years of age. The effect of age on dabigatran was also confirmed in a multivariate analysis of dabigatran concentrations versus ischemic and bleeding outcomes, where both age and renal clearance were found to be highly correlated predictive covariables.[31]

Rivaroxaban did not have a clinically significant increase in AUC in healthy elderly subjects of a pharmacokinetic study.[32] In the EINSTEIN VTE studies, there were no interactions between age and treatment effect for either recurrent VTE or "major or clinically relevant nonmajor bleeding."[15,16] When the 2 EINSTEIN studies were pooled and a nonpredefined new subgroup of "fragility" was created (defined by age >75 years, CrCl <50 mL/min, or body weight >50 kg), the authors did note a significant reduction in major bleeding (1.3% vs 4.5%), consistent with the pooled primary result.[14] With small numbers and the post hoc nature of the analysis, these data should be interpreted with caution. In ROCKET-AF, there were 6164 patients over age 75. Comparing rivaroxaban to VKA, the treatment effect in the subgroup greater than 75 was consistent with main trial findings: noninferior primary efficacy, noninferior major bleeding, and lower intracranial bleeding (all nonsignificant interactions). In contrast, older patients receiving rivaroxaban had higher rates of clinically relevant bleeding (interaction $P = .009$), largely driven by increased GI bleeding.[28]

For apixaban, there are no pharmacokinetic data available in healthy volunteers over age 75. An analysis of 768 patients over age 75 from the AMPLIFY VTE study (no dose adjustment) showed nonsignificant interaction and consistent results from the primary trial: noninferior efficacy and significantly reduced major bleeding.[18] In the ARISTOTLE study, apixaban-treated patients over age 80 who also either weighed 60 kg or less or had a serum creatinine of 1.5 mg/dL or greater had a 50% dose reduction.[19] In 5678 patients over age 75, there was a consistent treatment effect for higher primary efficacy, lower major bleeding, lower intracranial bleeding, and lower all bleeding (the relative effect of apixaban vs VKA was not modified by age for any of these endpoints).[33]

For edoxaban, there are no pharmacokinetic data available in healthy volunteers over age 75. There was prespecified dose reduction for patients with renal dysfunction, low body weight, or concomitant use of P-glycoprotein inhibitors, but no reduction based on age. In HOKUSAI-VTE study, there was a trend toward a greater reduction on the primary efficacy outcome for edoxaban versus VKA in 1104 elderly patients (interaction $P = .06$; 2.5% vs 5%). In terms of bleeding, edoxaban had a consistent effect in the elderly patient subgroup: less clinically major and clinically relevant nonmajor bleeding compared with VKA (nonsignificant interaction; 12.5% vs 15.1%). Major bleeding alone was not different in the primary trial and not analyzed in the elderly patient subgroup.[23] In ENGAGE AF-TIMI 48 study, high-dose edoxaban (60 mg daily in those without dose reduction) was comparable with VKA for the primary efficacy outcome, both in the overall trial and in 8474 elderly patients (nonsignificant interaction).[24] High-dose edoxaban was associated with less major bleeding, both in the overall trial and in the elderly patient subgroup (nonsignificant interaction). Although there was less intracranial bleeding ($P<.001$) and more GI bleeding ($P = .03$) for high-dose edoxaban 60 mg versus VKA in the primary trial, subgroup analyses were not reported for these secondary endpoints.

In conclusion, all current DOACs are associated with similar or better efficacy when compared with VKA in elderly patients. In terms of major bleeding risk, apixaban 5 mg and edoxaban 60 mg are safer than VKA in the elderly, whereas the relative safety of dabigatran 150 mg (vs VKA) in the elderly seems to be less favorable than in younger patients. Among all types of bleeding, intracranial bleeding is the most feared complication for any anticoagulant use in the elderly, because fatality rates are high even with available agents for rapid reversal in the case of VKA. Fortunately, available data suggest that nearly all DOACs at the currently approved doses (subgroup data for edoxaban not yet available but overall trial result is consistent with other DOACs) are associated with a lesser risk of intracranial bleeding when compared with VKA in

Table 3
DOAC use in elderly patients with age over 75: relative effects versus VKA in phase III trials

	Primary Efficacy, DOAC vs VKA	Major Bleeding, DOAC vs VKA	CNS Bleeding in AF, DOAC vs VKA	GI Bleeding in AF, DOAC vs VKA
Dabigatran 150 mg				
RECOVER I/II[10,29]	1.2 vs 1.8%/study (RR, 0.66; 95% CI 0.16–2.66)	3.5 vs 3.8%/study[d] (RR, 0.90; 95% CI 0.35–2.32)	n.r.	n.r.
RE-LY[12,29]	1.4 vs 2.1%/y (RR, 0.66; 95% CI 0.49–0.90)	5.1 vs 4.4%/y (RR, 1.18; 95% CI 0.98–1.42)[e]	0.4 vs 1.0%/y (RR, 0.42; 95% CI 0.25–0.70)	2.8 vs 1.6%/y (RR, 1.79; 95% CI 1.35–2.37)[f]
Interpretation	Lower stroke/SE and noninferior recurrent VTE	Trend toward higher bleeding	Lower bleeding	Higher bleeding
Rivaroxaban 20 mg				
EINSTEIN-DVT/PE[14,29]	2.3 vs 3.7%/study (RR, 0.62; 95% CI 0.33–1.18)	1.2 vs 4.5%/study (RR, n.r.; P sig)	n.r.	n.r.
ROCKET-AF[a,28]	2.3 vs 2.9%/y (RR, 0.80; 95% CI 0.63–1.02)	4.9 vs 4.4%/y (RR, 1.11; 95% CI 0.92–1.34)	0.7 vs 0.8%/y (RR, 0.80; 95% CI 0.50–1.28)	2.8 vs 1.7%/y (RR, n.r.; P = .0002)[g]
Interpretation	Noninferior recurrent VTE and stroke/SE	Noninferior bleeding	Lower bleeding[j]	Higher bleeding

Apixaban 5 mg				
AMPLIFY[18,29]	1.8 vs 3.6%/study (RR, 0.50; 95% CI 0.21–1.21)	1.0 vs 4.3%/study (RR, 0.27; 95% CI 0.11–0.66)		n.r.
ARISTOTLE[b,33]	1.6 vs 2.2%/y (RR, 0.71; 95% CI 0.53–0.95)	3.3 vs 5.2%/y (RR, 0.64; 95% CI 0.52–0.79)	0.4 vs 1.3%/y (RR, 0.34; 95% CI 0.20–0.57)	n.r.
Interpretation	Lower stroke/SE and noninferior recurrent VTE		Lower bleeding	
Edoxaban 60 mg				
HOKUSAI-VTE[c,23,29]	2.5 vs 5.0%/study (RR, 0.50; 95% CI 0.27–0.94)[h]	n.r.		n.r.
ENGAGE-AF-TIMI[c,24,29]	1.9 vs 2.3%/y (RR, 0.81; 95% CI 0.65–1.03)	4.0 vs 4.8%/y (RR, 0.81; 95% CI 0.67–0.98)		n.r.
Interpretation	Lower recurrent VTE and noninferior stroke/SE		Lower bleeding	

Abbreviations: AF, atrial fibrillation; DOAC, direct oral anticoagulants; n.r., not reported; NS, nonsignificant; RR, relative risk; SE, systemic embolism; sig, significant; VKA, vitamin K antagonist.

a Data interpretation according to the intention to treat analysis.

b Lower dose if 2 of the following: creatinine ≥1.5 mg/dL, age ≥80, or body weight ≤60 kg.

c Lower dose if any of the following: estimated creatinine clearance 30 to 50, BW ≤60, or verapamil/quinidine/dronedarone (P-glycoprotein inhibitors).

d Significant interaction between treatment and age for indicated subgroup (interaction P = .01).

e Significant interaction between treatment and age for indicated subgroup (interaction P<.001).

f Significant interaction between treatment and age for indicated subgroup (interaction P = .06).

g Significant interaction between treatment and age for indicated subgroup (interaction P = .009).

h Significant interaction between treatment and age for indicated subgroup (interaction P = .06).

i Interpretation (lower bleeding risk) extrapolated from the primary trial as the interaction term was nonsignificant.

the elderly. Interestingly, dabigatran 150 mg, rivaroxaban 20 mg, and edoxaban 60 mg seem to cause more GI bleeding than VKA in the overall population and the first 2 DOACs are also associated with more GI bleeding in the elderly. Thus, appropriate caution is warranted for use of DOACs in elderly patients with known risk factors for GI bleeding.

PATIENTS WITH MODERATE OR SEVERE RENAL IMPAIRMENT

Patients with kidney disease are not only at increased risk for thrombotic events,[34] they are often also at increased risk for major anticoagulant-related bleeding because of concomitant medications and/or underlying platelet dysfunction. DOACs must be selected and used with extra caution in this population because DOACs depend—to different degrees—on renal clearance. Nearly all of the large phase III trials involving DOACs have excluded patients with an eCrCl (as calculated by Cockcroft-Gault equation) of less than 30 mL/min (apixaban trials used eCrCl 25 as cutoff); thus, any dose recommendation in patients whose eCrCl is less than 30 mL/min is based on pharmacokinetic modelling rather than clinical outcomes. In a metaanalysis using phase III trial data, Harel and colleagues[35] found that DOACs, as a group, were noninferior to VKA for efficacy and bleeding in patients with moderate renal impairment (eCrCl, 30–50 mL/min). In this section, we compare each DOAC with VKA for the primary efficacy and "major bleeding" outcomes in patients with moderate renal impairment subgroup (**Table 4**). We will also present the data that led to currently FDA-approved dosing for severe renal impairment (**Table 5**).

Dabigatran is 80% renally excreted.[36] In patients with moderate renal impairment (eCrCl, 30–50 mL/min), administration of dabigatran 150 mg led to a 3.2 times higher AUC and a nonsignificant difference in maximum concentration (compared with healthy subjects).[36] In the pooled RECOVER studies where 245 patients had moderate renal impairment, there was no significant difference in primary efficacy or major bleeding for dabigatran versus VKA (nonsignificant interaction).[10] In a RE-LY subgroup analysis of 3505 patients who had an eCrCl of 30 to 50 mL/min (calculated by Cockcroft-Gault equation), dabigatran 150 mg was associated with improved primary efficacy and noninferior major bleeding compared with VKA, consistent with the primary trial effect (nonsignificant interaction).[12] However, when the same data were analyzed using Chronic Kidney Disease Epidemiology Collaboration formula for eCrCl, there was a significant interaction between eCrCl as a continuous variable and relative risk of major bleeding (interaction $P = .01$) such that there was a trend toward a greater number of major bleeding events with dabigatran 150 mg (vs VKA) at an eCrCl of less than 50 (HR, 1.22; 0.95–1.58).[37] In volunteers with severe renal dysfunction (eCrCl, 15–30 mL/min), dabigatran significantly increased the AUC (6.3 times), maximum concentration (2.1 times), and half-life (28 vs 14 hours) in comparison with patients with normal renal function.[36] Although not tested in clinical studies, the FDA approved a reduced dabigatran dose (75 mg bid) for AF patients with eCrCl 15 to 30 mL/min. Dabigatran is contraindicated in patients with eCrCl less than 15 mL/min and in patients on hemodialysis.

Approximately 30% of rivaroxaban elimination is renal.[38] In patients with moderate renal impairment (eCrCl, 30–50 mL/min), administration of rivaroxaban 10 mg led to a 1.5 times higher AUC and no difference in maximum concentration compared with healthy subjects.[39] In 633 patients with moderate renal insufficiency from the EINSTEIN studies, rivaroxaban was associated with noninferior primary efficacy (nonsignificant interaction) and lower major bleeding outcomes (unclear if significant interaction)[14]; however, as mentioned this is a subgroup of a subgroup analysis

Table 4
DOAC use in patients with moderate renal insufficiency (eCrCl 30–50 mL/min) calculated using Cockcroft-Gault equation: relative effects versus VKA in phase III trials

	Primary Efficacy, DOAC vs VKA	Major Bleeding, DOAC vs VKA
Dabigatran 150 mg		
RECOVER I/II (VTE)[10,35]	0 vs 3.9%/study (NS)	6.7 vs 2.9%/study (NS)[h]
RE-LY (AF)[11,12,37]	1.5 vs 2.8%/y (RR, 0.37; 95% CI 0.28–0.49)	5.4 vs 5.4%/y (RR, 0.97; 95% CI 0.78–1.19)
Interpretation	Lower stroke/SE and noninferior recurrent VTE	Noninferior with Cockcroft-Gault (trend toward higher bleeding with CKD-EPI)
Rivaroxaban 20 mg		
EINSTEIN-DVT/PE[14]	3.3 vs 3.4%/study (NS)	0.9 vs 4.1%/study (sig)
ROCKET-AF[a,17,35]	2.7 vs 3.1%/y (RR, 0.88; 95% CI 0.65–1.19)	3.4 vs 3.5%/y (RR, 0.97; 95% CI 0.74–1.27)
Interpretation	Noninferior stroke/SE and recurrent VTE	Noninferior bleeding
Apixaban 5 mg		
AMPLIFY (VTE)[18]	4.1 vs 4.4%/study (NS)	2.9 vs 5.5%/study (NS)[g]
ARISTOTLE (AF)[b,19,35]	2.1 vs 2.7%/y (RR, 0.79; 95% CI 0.56–1.12)[f]	3.2 vs 6.4%/y (RR, 0.52; 95% CI 0.40–0.68)[d]
Interpretation	Lower stroke/SE and noninferior recurrent VTE	Lower bleeding more pronounced in moderate renal impairment subgroup
Edoxaban 60 mg		
HOKUSAI-VTE[c,23]	3.0 vs 5.9%/study (NS)	n.r.
ENGAGE-AF-TIMI[c,24]	2.3 vs 2.7%/y (NS)[i]	3.1 vs 4.9%/y (sig)[e,i]
Interpretation	Noninferior stroke/SE and recurrent VTE	Lower bleeding more pronounced in the dose-adjusted subgroup

Abbreviations: AF, atrial fibrillation; CKD-EPI, Chronic Kidney Disease Epidemiology Collaboration; DOAC, direct oral anticoagulant; eCrCl, estimated creatinine clearance; n.r., not reported; NS, nonsignificant; SE, systemic embolism; sig, significant, VTE, venous thromboembolism.

[a] Data interpretation according to the intention to treat analysis, percent per year is calculated by dividing reported event rate over median follow-up of study.

[b] Lower dose if 2 of the following: creatinine ≥1.5 mg/dL, age ≥80, or body weight ≤60 kg.

[c] Lower dose if any of the following: eCrCl 30 to 50 mL/min, body weight ≤60, or verapamil/quinidine/dronedarone (P-glycoprotein inhibitors).

[d] Significant interaction between treatment and age for indicated subgroup (interaction P values = .03).

[e] Significant interaction between treatment and age for indicated subgroup (interaction P values = .02).

[f] Nonsignificant interactions (interaction P values = .72).

[g] Nonsignificant interactions (interaction P values = .36).

[h] Major bleeding data reported from RECOVER I study only (data not available from RECOVER II).

[i] Data extrapolated from "dose adjusted" subgroup for which 77% have eCrCl ≤50 mL/min.

thus the data is difficult to interpret. In 2949 patients with moderate renal impairment in the ROCKET-AF study, there was no difference (vs VKA) in primary efficacy or major bleeding outcomes, consistent with the primary trial result (nonsignificant interaction). Pharmacokinetic studies of patients with severe renal dysfunction (eCrCl, <30 mL/min), indicate that rivaroxaban AUC (1.6 times) and maximum concentration

Table 5
DOAC use in patients with renal impairment: FDA approved dosing based on eCrCl calculated using Cockcroft-Gault equation

	eCrCl >50 mL/min (Normal to Mild)	eCrCl 30–50 mL/min (Moderate)	eCrCl 15–30 mL/min (Severe)	eCrCl <15 mL/min (ESRD/HD)
Dabigatran				
VTE	150 mg bid	150 mg bid	No data[c]	No data[c]
AF	150 mg bid	150 mg bid	75 mg bid (PK data only)[c]	No data[c]
Rivaroxaban				
VTE	15 mg bid × 21 d then 20 mg qd	15 mg bid × 21 d then 20 mg qd	Avoid use[c]	Avoid use[c]
AF	20 mg qd	15 mg qd	15 mg qd (PK data only)[c]	Avoid use[c]
Apixaban				
VTE	10 mg bid × 7 d then 5 mg bid	10 mg bid × 7 d then 5 mg bid	No data[c]	No data[c]
AF	5 mg bid[a]	5 mg bid[a]	5 mg bid (PK data only)[a]	5 mg bid (PK data only)[a,c]
Edoxaban				
VTE	60 mg qd[b]	30 mg qd	30 mg qd (PK data only)	Avoid use
AF	60 mg qd[b] (avoid if CrCl >95 mL/min)	30 mg qd	30 mg qd (PK data only)	Avoid use

Abbreviations: AF, atrial fibrillation; bid, twice daily; CrCl, creatinine clearance; DOAC, direct oral anticoagulant; eCrCl, estimated creatinine clearance; ESRD/HD, end-stage renal disease/hemodialysis; FDA, US Food and Drug Administration; n.r., not reported; PK, pharmacokinetic; qd, daily; VKA, vitamin K antagonist; VTE, venous thromboembolism.
[a] Lower dose if 2 of the following: Cr ≥1.5 mg/dL, age ≥80, or BW ≤60 kg.
[b] Lower dose if any of the following: eCrCl 30 to 50 mL/min, BW ≤60, verapamil/quinidine/dronedarone (P-glycoprotein inhibitors).
[c] Use not recommended according to Health Canada labeling.

(1.3 times), and half-life (9.5 vs 8.3) are increased compared with healthy controls.[39] The FDA has approved 15 mg (reduced from 20 mg) daily for AF patients with eCrCl of 15 to 50 mL/min. Rivaroxaban is also contraindicated in patients with eCrCl of less than 15 mL/min or on hemodialysis.

The need for caution with dabigatran or rivaroxaban in patients with severe kidney disease is highlighted by a cohort study of 29,977 hemodialysis patients with AF. Despite the contraindication to dabigatran or rivaroxaban use in such patients, 5.9% of that patients in this cohort started 1 of these 2 DOACs between 2010 and 2014. Although the groups had different baseline characteristics, the adjusted survival analysis indicated that prescribing dabigatran or rivaroxaban rather than VKA to hemodialysis patients was associated with more major and fatal bleeding events.[40]

Apixaban is 27% renally excreted.[41] All clinical trials of apixaban excluded patients with an eCrCl less than of 25 mL/min. In AMPLIFY, there was no prespecified dose reduction based on eCrCl. In a subgroup analysis of 338 patients with moderate renal impairment, apixaban was noninferior to standard therapy for primary efficacy and associated with a numeric trend toward fewer major bleeding outcomes; both comparisons were consistent with the primary trial result (nonsignificant interactions).[18] In ARISTOTLE, there was a prespecified dose reduction for patients with a creatinine of

1.5 mg/dL or higher who also had either age 80 years or greater or a body weight of 60 kg or less. In a subgroup analysis of 3017 patients with moderate renal impairment, the relative treatment effect of apixaban versus VKA on the risk of stroke or systemic embolism was consistent with the results of the overall trial (nonsignificant interaction). For major bleeding, apixaban was even safer (vs VKA) in patients with moderate renal impairment than in those with normal renal function (interaction $P = .03$).[19] Severe renal impairment has also been studied in a pharmacokinetic data set of 16 patients. In this study, 8 end-stage renal disease subjects treated with a single dose of 5 mg apixaban had 36% higher AUC without dialysis and 4-hour hemodialysis decreased that exposure by 14% resulting in an overall 17% higher AUC in comparison with 8 healthy control subjects (NCT01340586).[40] The study did not examine the impact of subsequent or multiple doses of apixaban. Although the FDA adopted the labeling change to include dosing recommendation for nonvalvular AF patients with end-stage renal disease on hemodialysis in early 2014 (similar adjustment as those with moderate renal impairment), other agencies (including Health Canada) were less enthusiastic given the lack of clinical data to suggest efficacy or safety. Based on currently available data, apixaban, when used according to dose adjustments from the randomized trials, seems to have a safety profile that is particularly advantageous for patients with mild to moderate renal impairment. However, we suggest that apixaban (like other DOACs) should be avoided in patients with severe renal impairment or those with end-stage renal disease until more clinical outcome data are available.

Edoxaban is 50% renally excreted.[42] In both the HOKUSAI-VTE and ENGAGE AF-TIMI 48 trials, patients were excluded for an eCrCl of less than 30 mL/min and were given one-half the study dose for an eCrCl of less than 50 mL/min. In 540 patients with moderate renal impairment, subgroup analysis from HOKUSAI-VTE trial showed a nonsignificant difference in recurrent VTE/death, consistent with the primary result.[23] Major bleeding was no different in the primary trial and not reported in the subgroup with renal impairment. In ENGAGE AF-TIMI trial, moderate renal impairment contributed to approximately 76% (4074 of 5356) of edoxaban dose reduction. For stroke and systemic embolism, there was a consistent treatment effect in the dose-reduced subgroup (renal impairment was not reported as an isolated subgroup) for edoxaban 60 mg compared with VKA (nonsignificant interaction). For major bleeding, there was a significant further reduction of bleeding in the dose-reduced subgroups for high-dose edoxaban compared with VKA (interaction $P = .02$).[24] In AF patients with an eCrCl of 15 to 30 mL/min, preliminary evidence suggests that edoxaban 15 mg once daily achieves drug exposure and biomarker profiles similar to what one would expect with higher doses of edoxaban in patients with normal renal function.[43,44] Currently, the FDA-approved prescribing information recommends 30 mg rather than 15 mg once daily for patients with an eCrCl of between 15 and 50 mL/min and provides no guidance for patients with an eCrCl of less than 15 mL/min. Finally, edoxaban is contraindicated in patients with an eCrCl of greater than 95 mL/min because a post hoc analysis of the ENGAGE AF-TIMI 48 study showed that this subgroup of patients may have higher rates of ischemic stroke or systemic embolism with edoxaban 60 mg compared with VKA.[45]

In summary, the DOACs (as a class) seem to be at least as safe and effective as VKA in patients with moderate renal impairment (eCrCl, 30–50 mL/min). The degree to which individual DOACs depend on renal clearance varies; some DOACs (ie, apixaban and edoxaban) may be safer than VKA in patients with moderate renal impairment. At this time, there is no high-quality evidence to support DOAC use in patients with severe renal impairment (ie, those with eCrCl <15 mL/min or receiving renal replacement therapy). Enrollment of patients with end-stage renal disease in clinical trials of DOACs is encouraged.

PATIENTS WITH CANCER

Patients with cancer have a 4- to 7-fold higher risk of VTE in comparison with the general population.[46] Whereas low-molecular-weight heparin (LMWH) is the current standard of care treatment for cancer patients with VTE,[47] DOACs—if proven to be at least as safe and effective as LMWH in this population—would offer an attractive alternative because they would eliminate the need for hundreds of subcutaneous injections and they would lower the financial cost of treating cancer-associated VTE.

All of the phase III trials of DOACs for VTE have enrolled mostly noncancer patients, although some have included small numbers of cancer patients (see **Table 1**). In a metaanalysis of data from cancer patients who were enrolled in RCTs (n = 1132), Vedovati and colleagues[48] included 2 trials with dabigatran (RECOVER I & II), 2 with rivaroxaban (EINSTEIN-DVT & -PE), one with apixaban (AMPLIFY), and one with edoxaban (HOKUSAI). The authors concluded that DOACs are not significantly different in terms of efficacy (3.9% vs 6.0% VTE recurrence; OR, 0.63; 95% CI, 0.37–1.10) or safety (3.2% vs 4.2% major bleeding; OR 0.77 [95% CI, 0.41–1.44]) when compared with a treatment strategy mostly based on anticoagulation with VKA.

While this subgroup analysis is encouraging, there are several reasons that the use of DOACs for cancer-associated VTE should be restricted to clinical trials pending further evidence. First, the absolute rates of VTE recurrence among cancer patients from the DOAC trials are more than 50% lower than the corresponding rates documented in previously published studies that have established the superior efficacy of LMWH.[47] The lower recurrence rate among cancer patients in the DOAC trials raises the concern that very few patients with advanced or highly prothrombotic cancer were included in the DOAC VTE treatment trials. Second, the main comparator against which DOACs have been tested is VKA, a treatment strategy known to be less effective than LMWH in cancer-associated VTE. Third, other challenges faced by some cancer patients on active chemotherapy, such as unreliable oral absorption, variable drug clearance, thrombocytopenia, and drug–drug interactions (p-GP or CYP-3A4 inducers and inhibitors) highlight the importance of conducting dedicated clinical outcomes studies before drawing conclusions about the safety and efficacy of any anticoagulant in the treatment of cancer-associated VTE.

In conclusion, although the existing data are inadequate to recommend DOACs for the routine treatment or prevention of cancer-associated VTE, there are several ongoing clinical trials that may inform future clinical practice (**Table 6**). Enrollment in trials that compare DOACs directly with LMWH is recommended.

PATIENTS KNOWN TO HAVE THROMBOPHILIA OTHER THAN CANCER

In addition to cancer patients, several other populations are known to have high thrombophilic risk. In patients with mechanical heart valves, the use of dabigatran was associated with higher thromboembolic as well as bleeding complications in comparison with VKA.[49] The authors postulated that VKA might be more effective in suppressing the coagulation activation due to its effect on both the intrinsic (IX), extrinsic (VII), as well as common (X, II) pathways. The result of this study raises the important question whether other special populations who also possess high thrombophilic risks should avoid DOACs until proven otherwise.

One such population may be patients with APS, an autoimmune disease that causes systemic arterial and venous thrombosis. VKA with goal international normalized ratio of 2 to 3 is the current treatment recommendation for patients

Table 6
Ongoing clinical trials comparing DOACs versus standard treatment in cancer and APS patients

Trial	DOAC	Comparator	Population	Design	Enrollment
NCT02073682	Edoxaban	Dalteparin	Treatment of cancer-associated VTE	Phase III open-label RCT	3/2015
NCT01989845	Rivaroxaban	Historical control	Treatment of cancer-associated VTE in Asian patients	Phase II open-label prospective cohort	10/2013
NCT01708850 "Catheter 2"	Rivaroxaban	Historical control	Treatment of CVC-associated DVT in cancer patients	Phase II open-label prospective cohort	11/2012
NCT02048865 "AVERT"	Apixaban	Placebo	Prophylaxis of VTE in high-risk ambulatory cancer patients	Phase II double blind RCT	1/2014
NCT02066454 "MYELAXAT"	Apixaban	Historical control	Prophylaxis of VTE in myeloma patients treated with IMiD	Phase III open-label prospective cohort	4/2014
ISRCTN68222801 "RAPS"	Rivaroxaban	Warfarin	Treatment of VTE in APS patients	Phase II/III open-label RCT	11/2012
NCT02157272 "TRAPS"	Rivaroxaban	Warfarin	Treatment of VTE in triple-positive APS patients	Phase III open-label RCT	12/2014
NCT02116036 "RAPS"	Rivaroxaban	Historical control	Treatment of VTE in APS patients	Phase II open-label prospective cohort	9/2014

Abbreviations: APS, antiphospholipid antibody syndrome; CVC, central venous catheter; DOAC, direct oral anticoagulant; RCT, randomized, controlled trial; VTE, venous thromboembolism.

with APS-associated venous thrombosis.[50] However, many patients with APS develop recurrent VTE episodes while receiving VKA and it is challenging to determine the next step in management. There are several case reports of DOACs for treatment of APS with conflicting results. In 1 cohort of 26 patients with APS who had received either dabigatran or rivaroxaban, the event-free survival rate was 87.9% at 12 months with a median follow-up of 19 months, and there was 1 recurrent VTE and 2 bleeding events.[51] To the contrary, there were case reports where all APS patients on dabigatran or rivaroxaban had developed recurrent arterial or venous thrombosis.[52,53] Recently, the first RCT comparing rivaroxaban versus warfarin in patients with APS and prior VTE was completed after enrollment of 156 patients and the primary results, as measured by endogenous thrombin potential, were presented at the International Society on Thrombosis and Haemostasis 2015 meeting.[54] Currently, there are 2 open clinical trials evaluating the role of DOACs in APS (see **Table 6**). As with other areas of uncertainty with DOACs, enrollment in clinical trials is encouraged.

SUMMARY

Currently available evidence suggests that at least some of the DOACs—possibly at "adjusted" doses—will be an option for some patients with advanced age, extremes of body weight or impaired renal function. Although more than 100,000 patients were enrolled in the various DOAC registration trials, the relative safety and efficacy of DOACs in some situations (eg, patients with cancer, body weight >120 kg or eCrCl <15 mg/mL) will remain uncertain until more published evidence is available. Finally, because of the differences among DOACs in their dosing schemes, oral bioavailability, and routes of metabolism, each DOAC should be evaluated individually (including any recommended dose adjustment) when making decisions about the best anticoagulation strategy for a given patient in each clinical setting.

REFERENCES

1. Stein PD, Beemath A, Olson RE. Obesity as a risk factor in venous thromboembolism. Am J Med 2005;118:978–80.
2. Eichinger S, Hron G, Bialonczyk C, et al. Overweight, obesity, and the risk of recurrent venous thromboembolism. Arch Intern Med 2008;168:1678–83.
3. Guglin M, Maradia K, Chen R, et al. Relation of obesity to recurrence rate and burden of atrial fibrillation. Am J Cardiol 2011;107:579–82.
4. Pradaxa [package insert]. Ridgefield, CT: Boehringer Ingelheim Pharmaceuticals Inc; 2015.
5. Kubitza D, Becka M, Zuehlsdorf M, et al. Body weight has limited influence on the safety, tolerability, pharmacokinetics, or pharmacodynamics of rivaroxaban (BAY 59-7939) in healthy subjects. J Clin Pharmacol 2007;47:218–26.
6. Upreti VV, Wang J, Barrett YC, et al. Effect of extremes of body weight on the pharmacokinetics, pharmacodynamics, safety and tolerability of apixaban in healthy subjects. Br J Clin Pharmacol 2013;76:908–16.
7. Lip GY, Agnelli G. Edoxaban: a focused review of its clinical pharmacology. Eur Heart J 2014;35:1844–55.
8. Di Minno MN, Lupoli R, Di Minno A, et al. Effect of body weight on efficacy and safety of direct oral anticoagulants in the treatment of patients with acute venous thromboembolism: a meta-analysis of randomized controlled trials. Ann Med 2015;47:61–8.
9. Schulman S, Kearon C, Kakkar AK, et al. Dabigatran versus warfarin in the treatment of acute venous thromboembolism. N Engl J Med 2009;361:2342–52.
10. Schulman S, Kakkar AK, Goldhaber SZ, et al. Treatment of acute venous thromboembolism with dabigatran or warfarin and pooled analysis. Circulation 2014; 129:764–72.
11. Connolly SJ, Ezekowitz MD, Yusuf S, et al. Dabigatran versus warfarin in patients with atrial fibrillation. N Engl J Med 2009;361:1139–51.
12. Eikelboom JW, Wallentin L, Connolly SJ, et al. Risk of bleeding with 2 doses of dabigatran compared with warfarin in older and younger patients with atrial fibrillation. Circulation 2011;123:2363–72.
13. Ezekowitz ME, Parise H, Connolly SJ, et al. The use of dabigatran according to body mass index: the RE-LY experience. Eur Heart J 2014;35:1111.
14. Prins MH, Lensing AW, Bauersachs R, et al. Oral rivaroxaban versus standard therapy for the treatment of symptomatic venous thromboembolism: a pooled analysis of the EINSTEIN-DVT and PE randomized studies. Thromb J 2013;11:21.
15. Bauersachs R, Berkowitz SD, Brenner B, et al. Oral rivaroxaban for symptomatic venous thromboembolism. N Engl J Med 2010;363:2499–510.

16. Buller HR, Prins MH, Lensin AW, et al. Oral rivaroxaban for the treatment of symptomatic pulmonary embolism. N Engl J Med 2012;366:1287–97.

17. Patel MR, Mahaffey KW, Garg J, et al. Rivaroxaban versus warfarin in nonvalvular atrial fibrillation. N Engl J Med 2011;365:883–91.

18. Agnelli G, Buller HR, Cohen A, et al. Oral apixaban for the treatment of acute venous thromboembolism. N Engl J Med 2013;369:799–808.

19. Granger CB, Alexander JH, McMurray JJ, et al. Apixaban versus warfarin in patients with atrial fibrillation. N Engl J Med 2011;365:981–92.

20. Sandhu RK, Ezekowitz J, Andersson U, et al. The 'obesity paradox' in atrial fibrillation: observations from the ARISTOTLE (Apixaban for Reduction in Stroke and Other Thromboembolic Events in Atrial Fibrillation) trial. Eur Heart J 2016 Apr 12.

21. Yamashita T, Koretsune Y, Yasaka M, et al. Randomized, multicenter, warfarin-controlled phase II study of edoxaban in Japanese patients with non-valvular atrial fibrillation. Circ J 2012;76:1840–7.

22. Chung N, Jeon HK, Lien LM, et al. Safety of edoxaban, an oral factor Xa inhibitor, in Asian patients with non-valvular atrial fibrillation. Thromb Haemost 2011;105:535–44.

23. Buller HR, Décousus H, Grosso MA, et al. Edoxanban versus warfarin for the treatment of symptomatic venous thromboembolism. N Engl J Med 2013;369:1406–15.

24. Giugliano RP, Ruff CT, Braunwald E, et al. Edoxaban versus warfarin in patients with atrial fibrillation. N Engl J Med 2013;369:2093–104.

25. Breuer L, Ringwald J, Schwab S, et al. Ischemic stroke in an obese patient receiving dabigatran. N Engl J Med 2013;368:2440–2.

26. Anderson FA, Spencer FA. Risk factors for venous thromboembolism. Circulation 2003;107:I9–16.

27. Miyasaka Y, Barnes ME, Gersh BJ, et al. Secular trends in incidence of atrial fibrillation in Olmsted County, Minnesota, 1980 to 2000, and implications on the projections for future prevalence. Circulation 2006;114:119–25.

28. Halperin JL, Hankey GJ, Wojdyla DM, et al. Efficacy and safety of rivaroxaban compared with warfarin among elderly patients with nonvalvular atrial fibrillation in the rivaroxaban once daily, oral, direct factor Xa inhibition compared with vitamin K antagonism for prevention of stroke and embolism trial in atrial fibrillation (ROCKET AF). Circulation 2014;130:138–46.

29. Sharma M, Cornelius VR, Patel JP, et al. Efficacy and harms of direct oral anticoagulants in the elderly for stroke prevention in atrial fibrillation and secondary prevention of venous thromboembolism: systematic review and meta-analysis. Circulation 2015;132:194–204.

30. Stangier J, Stähle H, Rathgen K, et al. Pharmacokinetics and pharmacodynamics of the direct oral thrombin inhibitor dabigatran in healthy elderly subjects. Clin Pharmacokinet 2008;47:47–59.

31. Reilly PA, Lehr T, Haertter S, et al. The effect of dabigatran plasma concentrations and patient characteristics on the frequency of ischemic stroke and major bleeding in atrial fibrillation patients: the RE-LY Trial (Randomized Evaluation of Long-term Anticoagulation Therapy). J Am Coll Cardiol 2014;63:321–8.

32. Kubitza D, Becka M, Roth A, et al. The influence of age and gender on the pharmacokinetics and pharmacodynamics of rivaroxaban–an oral, direct Factor Xa inhibitor. J Clin Pharmacol 2013;53:249–55.

33. Halvorsen S, Atar D, Yang H, et al. Efficacy and safety of apixaban compared with warfarin according to age for stroke prevention in atrial fibrillation: Observations from the ARISTOTLE trial. Eur Heart J 2014;35:1864–72.
34. Olesen JB, Lip GY, Kamper AL, et al. Stroke and bleeding in atrial fibrillation with chronic kidney disease. N Engl J Med 2012;367:625–35.
35. Harel Z, Sholzberg M, Shah PS, et al. Comparisons between novel oral anticoagulants and vitamin K antagonists in patients with CKD. J Am Soc Nephrol 2014; 25:431–42.
36. Stangier J, Rathgen K, Stähle H, et al. The pharmacokinetics, pharmacodynamics and tolerability of dabigatran etexilate, a new oral direct thrombin inhibitor, in healthy male subjects. Br J Clin Pharmacol 2007;64:292–303.
37. Hijazi Z, Hohnloser SH, Oldgren J, et al. Efficacy and safety of dabigatran compared with warfarin in relation to baseline renal function in patients with atrial fibrillation: a RE-LY (randomized evaluation of long-term anticoagulation therapy) trial analysis. Circulation 2014;129:961–70.
38. Weinz C, Schwarz T, Kubitza D, et al. Metabolism and excretion of rivaroxaban, an oral, direct factor Xa inhibitor, in rats, dogs, and humans. Drug Metab Dispos 2009;37:1056–64.
39. Kubitza D, Becka M, Mueck W, et al. Effects of renal impairment on the pharmacokinetics, pharmacodynamics and safety of rivaroxaban, an oral, direct Factor Xa inhibitor. Br J Clin Pharmacol 2010;70:703–12.
40. Chan KE, Edelman ER, Wenger JB, et al. Dabigatran and rivaroxaban use in atrial fibrillation patients on hemodialysis. Circulation 2015;131:972–9.
41. Raghavan N, Frost CE, Yu Z, et al. Apixaban metabolism and pharmacokinetics after oral administration to humans. Drug Metab Dispos 2009;37:74–81.
42. Bathala MS, Masumoto H, Oguma T, et al. Pharmacokinetics, biotransformation, and mass balance of edoxaban, a selective, direct factor Xa inhibitor, in humans. Drug Metab Dispos 2012;40:2250–5.
43. Yin OQ, Tetsuya K, Miller R. Edoxaban population pharmacokinetics and exposure-response analysis in patients with non-valvular atrial fibrillation. Eur J Clin Pharmacol 2014;70:1339–51.
44. Koretsune Y, Yamashita T, Kimura T, et al. Short-term safety and plasma concentrations of edoxaban in Japanese patients with non-valvular atrial fibrillation and severe renal impairment. Circ J 2015;79:1486–95.
45. Savaysa [package insert]. Parsippany, NJ: Daiichi Sankyo Inc; 2015.
46. Heit JA, Silverstein MD, Mohr DN, et al. Risk factors for deep vein thrombosis and pulmonary embolism: a population-based case-control study. Arch Intern Med 2000;160:809–15.
47. Lee AY, Levine MN, Baker RI, et al. Low-molecular-weight heparin versus a coumarin for the prevention of recurrent venous thromboembolism in patients with cancer. N Engl J Med 2003;349:146–53.
48. Vedovati MC, Germini F, Agnelli G, et al. Direct oral anticoagulants in patients with VTE and cancer: a systematic review and meta-analysis. Chest 2015;147:475–83.
49. Eikelboom JW, Connolly SJ, Brueckmann M, et al. Dabigatran versus warfarin in patients with mechanical heart valves. N Engl J Med 2013;369:1206–14.
50. Giannakopoulos B, Krilis SA. How I treat the antiphospholipid syndrome. Blood 2009;114:2020–30.
51. Noel N, Dutasta F, Costedoat-Chalumeau N, et al. Safety and efficacy of oral direct inhibitors of thrombin and factor Xa in antiphospholipid syndrome. Autoimmun Rev 2015;14:680–5.

52. Schaefer JK, McBane RD, Black DF, et al. Failure of dabigatran and rivaroxaban to prevent thromboembolism in antiphospholipid syndrome: a case series of three patients. Thromb Haemost 2014;112:947–50.

53. Win K, Rodgers GM. New oral anticoagulants may not be effective to prevent venous thromboembolism in patients with antiphospholipid syndrome. Am J Hematol 2014;89:1017.

54. Cohen H, Doré CJ, Clawson S, et al. Rivaroxaban in antiphospholipid syndrome (RAPS) protocol: a prospective, randomized controlled phase II/III clinical trial of rivaroxaban versus warfarin in patients with thrombotic antiphospholipid syndrome, with or without SLE. Lupus 2015;24(10):1087–94.

Perioperative Management of the Direct Oral Anticoagulants: A Case-Based Review

Benjamin R. Bell, MD[a],*, Alex C. Spyropoulos, MD[b],
James D. Douketis, MD[c]

KEYWORDS

- Direct oral anticoagulants • Perioperative management • Algorithm • Thrombosis

KEY POINTS

- Not all procedures require anticoagulants to be held (eg, minor dental and skin procedures, cataract extraction, selected cardiac device implantation).
- Bridging anticoagulation does not seem to mitigate the risk for perioperative thromboembolism, but is associated with an increase in major bleeding; consequently, bridging anticoagulation is not routinely recommended for DOAC-treated patients during treatment interruption for an elective surgery/procedure.
- DOACs should be held for 1 to 4 days preprocedure, with the interruption interval depending on the DOAC, patient renal function, and surgery/procedure bleeding risk.
- Postoperative resumption of DOACs should take into account their rapid onset of action (1–3 hours postingestion), and can be restarted approximately 24 hours after low-bleed-risk and 48 to 72 hours after high-bleed-risk procedures.
- With urgent surgery, there is no evidence for more bleeding among DOAC-treated compared with warfarin-treated patients.

INTRODUCTION

There are an estimated 33.5 million people worldwide with atrial fibrillation (AF), and an additional 5 million cases are diagnosed annually.[1] Because AF is more common among the elderly, the North American incidence is expected to rise as the population ages.[2] Most patients with AF should receive an oral anticoagulant to prevent stroke, and practice guidelines recommend the direct oral anticoagulants (DOACs) in preference to warfarin.[3,4]

a University of Toronto, Toronto, Ontario, Canada; b Anticoagulation Services and Clinical Thrombosis Services, Northwell Health Systems at Lenox Hill Hospital, Hofstra Northwell School of Medicine, 130 E, 77th St., New York, NY 10075, USA; c Division of Hematology and Thromboembolism, Department of Medicine, McMaster University, St. Joseph's Hospital, 50 Charlton Avenue East, Room F-544, Hamilton, ON L8N 4A6, Canada
* Corresponding author. North York General Hospital, 4001 Leslie Street, Willowdale, Ontario M2K 1E1, Canada.
E-mail address: ben.bell@nygh.on.ca

Hematol Oncol Clin N Am 30 (2016) 1073–1084
http://dx.doi.org/10.1016/j.hoc.2016.05.005
0889-8588/16/$ – see front matter © 2016 Elsevier Inc. All rights reserved.

Approximately 10% of patients on anticoagulants require treatment interruption annually for a surgery or invasive procedure.[5] It is important that such treatment interruptions balance the procedure-related bleeding risk against the patient's thrombotic risk. Thus, excess bleeding may occur if an anticoagulant is not interrupted soon enough or restarted too quickly postprocedure[6]; conversely, extended interruption of anticoagulants may expose patients to an increased risk for thrombotic complications.[7] Of concern, observational studies have shown that periprocedural management of anticoagulants is variable and often not in keeping with guideline recommendations.[8]

Clinical guidelines are available for the periprocedural management of warfarin (and other vitamin K antagonists) but are lacking for patients who are receiving DOACs, which comprise dabigatran, rivaroxaban, apixaban, and edoxaban.[9] There are key differences between the DOACs and warfarin related to elimination half-life (10–14 hours for DOACs vs 38–42 hours for warfarin), dependence on renal elimination (25%–75% renal clearance for DOACs vs nonrenal clearance for warfarin), and peak action after oral intake (1–3 hours for DOACs vs 4–6 days for warfarin), which necessitate different periprocedural management approaches.

Using a case-based approach, this article provides practical clinical guidance for the periprocedural management of patients who are receiving a DOAC and require an elective or urgent surgery/procedure. Current practice recommendations are based on low-quality evidence derived mainly from DOAC pharmacokinetic data (Table 1), retrospective studies, and patient registries.[10] However, there are emerging prospective studies assessing the safety of standardized periprocedural DOAC management protocols, including the one recommended in this text.[11] In addition, the PAUSE trial (NCT02228798) will assess standardized, DOAC-specific management protocols in approximately 3000 patients who are receiving a DOAC.

CASE 1: MINIMAL-BLEED-RISK PROCEDURE

A 78-year-old woman with AF, hypertension, mildly impaired left ventricular function, and a transient ischemic attack 7 months ago is scheduled to have multiple teeth extracted. Her estimated creatinine clearance is 56 mL/min. She takes rivaroxaban, 20 mg daily with breakfast, for stroke prevention. Her dentist asks you if the rivaroxaban can be continued through the procedure.

When considering withholding anticoagulants, one should balance the risk of bleeding associated with a procedure and the patient's risk for thromboembolic complications while off anticoagulants. Patients' risk for procedure-related bleeding is stratified as minimal, low, and high bleed risk based on observed bleeding rates postoperatively for patients not on anticoagulants (Table 2).[5] Neuraxial blocks or anesthesia are somewhat unique procedures because they are associated with a low

Table 1
Pharmacologic characteristics of the DOACs

Target	Dabigatran	Rivaroxaban	Apixaban	Edoxaban
	Factor IIa (Thrombin)	Factor Xa	Factor Xa	Factor Xa
Dosing (atrial fibrillation)	150 mg bid[a]	20 mg daily[b]	5 mg bid[c]	60 mg daily[d]
Cmax	1–2 h	2–4 h	3–4 h	1–2 h

[a] 110 mg bid if older than age 80 or if additional risk factors for bleeding.
[b] 15 mg od if creatinine clearance 30 to 50.
[c] 2.5 mg bid if two of the following: age greater than 80, serum creatinine greater than 133, weight less than 60 kg.
[d] 30 mg daily if creatinine clearance 30 to 50 or weight less than 60 kg.

Table 2
Bleeding risk associated with selected procedures

Procedural Bleeding Risk		
Minimal	**Low**	**High**

• Dental procedures
  ○ Up to two tooth
    extractions
  ○ Subgingival scaling
  ○ Gingival biopsy
  ○ Periodontal surgery
  ○ Root canal
• Minor skin procedures
  ○ Skin biopsy
  ○ Excision
• Cataract extraction
• Endoscopic procedures
  without biopsy
• Pacemaker/implantable
  cardioverter defibrillator
  implantation[a]
	• Laparoscopic
	  cholecystectomy
	• Laparoscopic inguinal
	  hernia repair
	• Other dermatologic
	  procedures
	• Noncataract
	  ophthalmologic
	  procedures
	• Coronary angiography
	• Other intra-abdominal,
	  intrathoracic, orthopedic,
	  or vascular surgery
		• Any procedure involving
		  neuraxial anesthesia
		• Neurosurgery (intracranial or
		  spinal surgery)
		• Cardiac surgery (eg, coronary
		  artery bypass graft, heart
		  valve replacement)
		• Major vascular surgery (eg,
		  aortic aneurysm repair,
		  aortofemoral bypass)
		• Major urologic surgery (eg,
		  prostatectomy, bladder
		  tumor resection)
		• Major lower limb orthopedic
		  surgery (eg, hip/knee joint
		  replacement surgery)
		• Lung resection surgery
		• Intestinal anastomosis
		• Selected procedures (eg,
		  kidney biopsy, prostate
		  biopsy, cervical cone biopsy,
		  pericardiocentesis, colonic
		  polypectomy)

[a] Refers to selected patients on warfarin; for patients on DOACs, alternate approaches may be equally reasonable.

absolute risk of bleeding but are managed as a high-bleed-risk procedure because of the potentially devastating consequence, namely lower limb paralysis, if epidural bleeding occurs.[12]

Data from randomized trials and observational studies involving the periprocedural management of patients on warfarin inform practice for patients undergoing minimal-bleed-risk procedures, including minor dental and dermatologic procedures, cataract extraction, and certain cardiac device procedures.[9] For patients on warfarin, not interrupting treatment is associated with a low risk of major and/or clinically relevant bleeding and thrombotic events. To address the excess bleeding observed with this strategy (eg, minor gingival mucosal bleeding, self-limited dermal bleeding, and subconjunctival hemorrhage), methods to optimize hemostasis include tranexamic acid mouthwash for gingival bleeding, and the use of prohemostatic sutures/cautery for dermatologic and cardiac device procedures.

For DOAC-treated patients, a similar strategy of continuing the anticoagulant around minimal-bleed-risk procedures is likely an acceptable option, although procedure-specific evidence is lacking. In a retrospective analysis of patients undergoing invasive procedures in the ARISTOTLE study, a randomized trial comparing apixaban with warfarin for stroke prevention in AF, there was no observed difference in periprocedural bleeding rates between warfarin- and apixaban-treated patients.[13] Notably, about 37% of patients from each group continued the anticoagulant through the procedure. Data from the RE-LY study, a randomized trial comparing dabigatran with warfarin for stroke prevention in AF, found that periprocedural bleeding rates were not significantly different between warfarin- and dabigatran-treated patients, although all patients studied interrupted anticoagulant therapy.[14] Similarly, in the ROCKET-AF trial, which compared rivaroxaban with warfarin for stroke prevention in AF, rates of periprocedural bleeding were comparable with interruption of warfarin and rivaroxaban.[15] Finally, real world data from the Dresden registry suggests a similar safety profile, including low bleeding and thrombotic risk, for continuing rivaroxaban through minimal and minor procedures.[16]

Returning to the case example, it is reasonable for this patient to continue DOAC treatment around the time of her procedure and, as a precaution, take tranexamic acid mouthwash just before and two to three times after the procedure. However, we suggest she delays taking rivaroxaban until after the procedure (ie, with dinner on the same day) because if rivaroxaban is taken in the morning, this would lead to a peak anticoagulant effect 1 to 3 hours after intake, which is close to the time of the procedure and may lead to excessive bleeding.

CASE 2: HIGH THROMBOTIC RISK

A 42-year-old obese man suffered an unprovoked pulmonary embolism (PE) 15 days ago. He has a history of recurrent biliary colic and had been scheduled to undergo an elective laparoscopic cholecystectomy, before the PE, 1 week from now. He is otherwise healthy, and his only medication is apixaban, 5 mg twice daily. The surgeon wants to know if a temporary inferior vena cava (IVC) filter or bridging anticoagulation should be used perioperatively.

As with warfarin-treated patients, patient-specific thrombotic risk should be considered (**Table 3**) before withholding a DOAC. In the case of urgent surgery, the risk

Table 3
Thrombotic risk stratification by indication for anticoagulant

	Indication for Anticoagulant		
Thromboembolic Risk	**Mechanical Valve[a]**	**Atrial Fibrillation**	**Venous Thromboembolism**
Low	Bileaflet aortic prosthesis without CHADS risk factors	CHADS 0–2 without previous stroke/TIA	VTE >12 mo prior
Moderate	Bileaflet aortic prosthesis with CHADS score of $\geq$1	CHADS 3–4	• VTE within the past 3–12 mo • Nonsevere thrombophilia • Recurrent VTE • Active cancer
High	• Any mitral prosthesis • Caged ball/tilting disk aortic prosthesis • Stroke/TIA in past 6 mo	• CHADS 5–6 • Previous stroke/TIA • Rheumatic valvular heart disease[a]	• VTE within last 3 mo • Severe thrombophilia[b]

Abbreviations: TIA, transient ischemic attack; VTE, venous thromboembolism.

[a] DOACs should not be used for patients with mechanical valves or rheumatic heart disease, where warfarin remains the standard of care.

[b] Severe thrombophilia includes homozygous factor V Leiden/prothrombin gene mutation, protein C/S deficiency, antiphospholipid antibodies.

Adapted from Douketis JD, Spyropoulos AC, Spencer FA, et al. Perioperative management of antithrombotic therapy: antithrombotic therapy and prevention of thrombosis, 9th ed: American College of Chest physicians evidence-based clinical practice guidelines. Chest 2012;141:e326S–50S.

associated with thrombosis, in general, is less than the risk associated with delaying surgery. However, in cases of elective surgery where an anticoagulant will be temporarily interrupted, this balance should be weighed accordingly.

Venous thromboembolism (VTE), which includes deep venous thrombosis and PE, is associated with the highest risk of clot extension, propagation, and embolism during the initial 4 weeks from the time of diagnosis, and is the period when anticoagulant interruption should be deferred if possible.[17] An IVC filter may prevent deep venous thrombosis embolization but is associated with an increased risk for recurrent deep venous thrombosis and does not affect mortality.[18] In general, an IVC filter is indicated for patients with acute VTE in whom there is a prolonged (>24 hour) contraindication to anticoagulation because of bleeding or need for an urgent surgery/procedure; IVC filters should not be used perioperatively for elective surgery. In the latter circumstances, surgery should be delayed for at least 1 month, and preferably for 3 months, after which time anticoagulation can be safely interrupted.[9,19,20]

Because of the pharmacokinetic similarities between the DOACs and low-molecular-weight heparins (LMWHs), with a rapid onset and rapid offset of action, the use of bridging anticoagulation is considered superfluous in DOAC-treated patients who need treatment interruption for an elective surgery/procedure.[21] In warfarin-treated patients, observational studies suggest that bridging confers an increased risk for perioperative bleeding.[22] The Dresden DOAC registry showed a 3.6-fold higher risk for major bleeding in bridged compared with not bridged patients.[16] Similarly, in a substudy of the RE-LY trial, which assessed patients who required warfarin or dabigatran interruption for a surgery/procedure, bridging anticoagulation was an independent risk factor for major bleeding in dabigatran-treated (odds ratio, 5.02) and warfarin-treated (odds ratio, 6.06) patients, with no observed reduction in thromboembolic events.[23]

The BRIDGE study, a randomized, placebo-controlled trial that compared bridging or no bridging strategies in warfarin-treated patients with AF who required an elective surgery/procedure, found that bridging anticoagulation conferred an approximately three-fold increased risk for major bleeding and did not mitigate the risk for thromboembolism.[24] Given the pharmacologic similarities between the DOACs and LMWHs, coupled with accumulating data suggesting harm with bridging anticoagulation, the totality of evidence argues against the use of bridging anticoagulation for patients on DOACs who require an elective surgery/procedure. However, postoperative use of prophylactic doses of LMWH may be considered for patients at high risk for VTE in whom intake of oral medications (including DOACs) is not possible (eg, postoperative ileus).

For the case example, we would defer elective surgery until at least 1 month and, ideally, 3 months of anticoagulant therapy for VTE is complete. We would not advise for the perioperative use of IVC filters for elective surgery, nor the use of bridging anticoagulation for DOAC-treated patients.

CASE 3: LOW-BLEED-RISK PROCEDURE

Following 3 months of anticoagulation with apixaban for an unprovoked PE, an otherwise healthy obese 42-year-old man is scheduled to undergo a laparoscopic cholecystectomy for recurrent biliary colic. His thrombosis specialist has recommended indefinite anticoagulation. His estimated creatinine clearance is greater than 60 mL/min. You are asked to manage his anticoagulation perioperatively.

Following a minimum 3 months of anticoagulant therapy from the time of diagnosis, it is reasonable to proceed with elective surgery in a patient with a history of VTE.

Unlike minimal-bleed-risk procedures, anticoagulant medications should be held perioperatively for patients undergoing low- or high-bleed-risk procedures (see **Table 2**). Guidance for the interruption period for DOACs before a surgery/procedure is based on DOAC half-lives, patient renal function, and surgery/procedure bleed risk (**Table 4**). For low-bleed-risk procedures DOACs should be withheld for a two- to three-drug half-life interval, whereas for high-bleed-risk procedures, this interval should be extended to allow a four to five half-life interval preprocedure.[5] Postoperative resumption should account for the rapid peak anticoagulant effect of DOACs that occurs 1 to 3 hours after ingestion and a suggested resumption schedule is provided (**Table 5**); however, there is a need to ensure hemostasis is secured before restarting therapeutic doses of a rapidly acting anticoagulant, such as a DOAC or LMWH. Assuming that the risk for thromboembolism is not very high, it is reasonable to use a lower, prophylactic dose of anticoagulants during the initial 24 to 72 hours after surgery (eg, dalteparin, 5000 IU daily; enoxaparin, 30 mg twice a day; dabigatran, 75–110 mg daily/twice a day; rivaroxaban, 10–15 mg daily; apixaban, 2.5 mg twice a day), before increasing to therapeutic doses. In general, one can resume treatment-dose DOAC therapy approximately 24 hours after a low-bleed-risk procedure, and 48 to 72 hours after high-bleed-risk procedure.

In a prospective cohort study of 541 dabigatran-treated patients with AF undergoing an elective surgery/procedure, a standardized perioperative management protocol seemed safe and effective, with low rates of thromboembolism (0.2%) and major bleeding (1.8%) at 30 days postprocedure.[11] Notably, 73% of patients had dabigatran resumed within 48 hours of the procedure. Such data are favorable when compared with perioperative outcomes observed in warfarin-treated patients.[25] In the RE-LY perioperative analysis, bleeding rates at 30 days were not statistically different among patients on dabigatran, 110 mg twice a day (3.8%); dabigatran, 150 mg twice a day (5.1%); or warfarin (4.6%).[14] While we await prospective validation of standardized perioperative management protocols for rivaroxaban- and apixaban-treated patients,

Table 4
Preoperative DOAC management based on drug half-life and surgical bleed risk

| | Interval Between Last DOAC Dose and Procedure[a] | |
| | Low-Bleed-Risk Procedure[b] | High-Bleed-Risk Procedure[b] |
Creatinine Clearance (mL/min)	2–3 Drug Half-Lives	4–5 Drug Half-Lives
Dabigatran		
>50	At least 24 h (skip 2 doses)	At least 48 h (skip 4 doses)
30–50	At least 48 h (skip 4 doses)	At least 96 h (skip 8 doses)
Rivaroxaban		
>50	At least 24 h (skip 1 dose)	At least 48 h (skip 2 doses)
30–50	At least 24 h (skip 1 dose)	At least 48 h (skip 2 doses)
Apixaban		
>50	At least 24 h (skip 2 doses)	At least 48 h (skip 4 doses)
25–50	At least 24 h (skip 2 doses)	At least 48 h (skip 4 doses)
Edoxaban		
>50	At least 24 h (skip 1 dose)	At least 48 h (skip 2 doses)
30–50	At least 24 h (skip 1 dose)	At least 48 h (skip 2 doses)

[a] DOAC not taken on day of surgery/procedure.
[b] See **Table 2** for procedural definitions.

Table 5
Suggested postoperative resumption protocol for the DOACs

	Resumption of DOAC After Surgery/Procedure	
DOAC	Low-Bleed-Risk	High-Bleed-Risk
Dabigatran	Resume AM postoperative day +1 (24 h)	Resume AM postoperative day +2 to +3 (48–72 h)
Rivaroxaban	As above	As above
Apixaban	As above	As above
Edoxaban	As above	As above

Note this is a suggested algorithm and therapeutic doses of anticoagulants should be started only after hemostasis is established. Consideration for thromboprophylactic or intermediate doses of anticoagulants in the first 24 to 72 hours following surgery can be considered (see text).

similar rates of bleeding and thromboembolism were observed in the DOAC and warfarin arms in patients who underwent invasive procedures in the ROCKET-AF (rivaroxaban vs warfarin in AF) and ARISTOTLE (apixaban vs warfarin in AF) trials.[13,15]

In a 2015 guideline statement by North American and European anesthesia societies, it was recommended that dabigatran be withheld for 4 to 6 days, rivaroxaban for 3 days, and apixaban for 3 to 5 days before a neuraxial procedure,[12] with LMWH bridging to be considered in patients at high risk for thrombosis. These interruption intervals assume the longest possible elimination half-life for each DOAC and may be excessive. Although we agree that the interruption interval of a DOAC and neuraxial analgesia/anesthesia should be based, in part, on the DOAC elimination half-life, what may be more useful to clinicians is the actual residual anticoagulant effect at the time of neuraxial procedure with standardized interruption protocols for each DOAC. This approach has been used to determine the interruption interval of warfarin, LMWHs, and unfractionated heparin before a surgery/neuraxial anesthesia and we suggest the same approach is used for DOACs. The PAUSE study (NCT02228798) plans to measure the residual anticoagulant effect of DOACs in approximately 1000 patients for each DOAC and aims to demonstrate that the proposed standardized anticoagulant interruption protocols result in a minimal to no residual anticoagulant effect before a high-bleed-risk procedure and/or neuraxial anesthesia. Additional studies are needed so that recommendations on DOAC interruption are based on the effects of standardized interruption protocols on clinical bleeding and residual anticoagulant effect.

In this case example, given the procedure bleed risk and patient creatinine clearance, the apixaban was held 24 hours before the elective laparoscopic cholecystectomy, and restarted at full dose on postoperative Day 1.

CASE 4: URGENT SURGERY

An 87-year-old woman presents to hospital with 36 hours of worsening abdominal pain. She is febrile, tachycardic, and hypotensive with peritoneal signs at initial assessment. Urgent computed tomography scan of the abdomen reveals a large bowel obstruction secondary to a sigmoid mass with perforation. She carries diagnoses of hypertension and AF, treated with perindopril, 8 mg daily, and dabigatran, 110 mg twice daily. Her lactate is 3.5 mmol/L, creatinine clearance is 42 mL/min, international normalized ratio is 1.2, and activated partial thromboplastin time (aPTT) is 36 seconds. She took her last dose of dabigatran 18 hours ago. Her surgeon wants to take her to the operating room as soon as possible for a Hartmann procedure. What is your management?

Optimizing a patient for urgent surgery on an anticoagulant medication would ideally involve knowing whether or not the anticoagulant is present, and rapidly reversing any residual effect. In warfarin-treated patients, this involves measuring the international normalized ratio and, if greater than 1.4, administering prothrombin complex concentrate and vitamin K intravenously.[26,27] Although there are coagulation tests that reliably measure the anticoagulant effect of dabigatran (dilute thrombin time) and oral factor Xa inhibitors (DOAC-calibrated anti-factor Xa levels), these tests are not yet widely available and the interpretation of test results, including definition of normal ranges, has not been standardized. Routinely available coagulation tests (eg, international normalized ratio, aPTT) may not provide reliable and precise measures of the anticoagulant effects of DOACs. For dabigatran, a normal thrombin time excludes dabigatran effect, but this test is overly sensitive to dabigatran's anticoagulant effect, and the thrombin time may be prolonged even with clinically insignificant dabigatran levels (**Table 6**). A normal aPTT has been suggested to exclude a clinically important dabigatran anticoagulant effect, but only if a highly sensitive aPTT assay is used.[28]

Delaying urgent surgery to allow for DOAC metabolism/excretion is advisable for patients in whom drug is expected to be present, based on time from last dose and drug half-life. If surgery cannot be delayed, the surgeon should expect excess hemorrhage. This is managed with prohemostatic agents (eg, four-factor prothrombin complex concentrate), supportive care (eg, intravenous fluids, red cell transfusion, platelet transfusion for patients on concomitant ASA/P2Y12 inhibitors), and intraoperative measures (eg, greater attention to blood vessel ligation/cautery).[29]

Despite the lack of a widely available reversal agent for the DOACs, hemorrhagic complications were no different between the warfarin and DOAC arms for patients undergoing urgent/emergent surgery in the RE-LY, ROCKET-AF, and ARISTOTLE trials.[13–15] However, urgent surgery was an independent predictor of major hemorrhage in the DOAC and warfarin arms, highlighting the morbidity associated with nonelective procedures.

Table 6
Interpretation of coagulation tests for patients treated with DOACs

	Dabigatran	Rivaroxaban	Apixaban
International normalized ratio/ prothrombin time		Elevated: drug present Normal: drug may be present	Not useful
aPTT	Elevated: drug present Normal: drug may be present		
Thrombin time	Elevated: drug present Normal: no drug present[b]		
Dilute thrombin time (Hemoclot)[a]	Elevated: drug present Normal: no significant drug present		
Calibrated anti-Xa[a]		Elevated: drug present Normal: no significant drug present	Elevated: drug present Normal: no significant drug present

[a] Not routinely available.
[b] Thrombin time may be elevated with clinically insignificant dabigatran levels.

Idarucizumab is a monoclonal antibody fragment with high affinity to dabigatran. It rapidly binds dabigatran and reverses its anticoagulant effect,[30] and has been approved for use in the United States and Canada. The REVERSE-AD cohort trial is investigating the efficacy and safety of idarucizumab, and is actively enrolling patients who require urgent surgery while on dabigatran, or have life-threatening bleeding while on dabigatran. Preliminary results from this study demonstrate that 92% of enrolled patients who required urgent surgery had normal intraoperative hemostasis, as judged by the surgeon.[31] Andexanet-a is a factor Xa decoy molecule that contains the rivaroxaban/apixaban binding site, but lacks the serine protease, so although it binds the anticoagulant it does not participate in the coagulation cascade.[32] Studies of andexanet-a in healthy volunteers taking apixaban or rivaroxaban demonstrate a normalization of anti-Xa levels with a bolus followed by an infusion of the reversal agent,[33] and a study in bleeding patients is ongoing (NCT02329327).

Despite normal routine coagulation parameters, the time from last ingestion and creatinine clearance would predict clinically relevant dabigatran levels in this patient. Therefore, she received idarucizumab preoperatively (two intravenous infusions of 2.5 g each). She was taken to the operating room where a locally advanced sigmoid carcinoma was observed. She underwent a peritoneal washout and Hartmann procedure. Normal intraoperative and postoperative hemostasis was noted by the surgeon. She experienced a postoperative ileus, so prophylactic dosing of dalteparin (5000 units subcutaneously once daily) was started 48 hours after surgery. She was switched back to dabigatran, 110 mg orally twice daily, once her ileus resolved and additional invasive procedures were not planned.

SUMMARY

The periprocedural management of patients on DOACs is a common clinical problem but prospective data to inform best practices are lacking. Retrospective analyses from randomized trials and patient registry data suggest that the DOACs are easily managed in a manner that does not result in excess hemorrhage or thrombosis. Assessment of procedural bleeding risk is always the first step, and the clinician must remember that not all procedures necessitate a temporary interruption of anticoagulant medications. For example, up to two tooth extractions, skin biopsies, and cataract extraction can generally be done safely without interrupting DOACs.

Patient-specific thrombotic risk also must be considered. Generally speaking, however, bridging anticoagulation is not indicated for patients treated with DOACs because of mounting evidence of harm caused by excess bleeding without thromboembolic benefit. If the anticoagulant is to be held, the clinician should consider the pharmacokinetic properties of DOACs, patient renal function, and surgical bleed risk as factors to determine the appropriate duration of preoperative interruption and postoperative resumption of anticoagulant therapy. Given their rapid onset of action, the DOACs should not be restarted postoperatively at full dose until hemostasis has been established. Consideration can be given to thromboprohylaxis with LMWH, or a DOAC, in the first 24 to 72 hours postoperatively.

Additional studies are needed to inform best practices. In the meantime, standardized approaches to the perioperative anticoagulant management are available that are based on the available evidence. The algorithm presented in this article is available *free of charge* at the Thrombosis Canada Web site at http://thrombosiscanada.ca in app, tool, and text format.

REFERENCES

1. Chugh SS, Havmoeller R, Narayanan K, et al. Worldwide epidemiology of atrial fibrillation: a Global Burden of Disease 2010 Study. Circulation 2014;129:837–47.
2. Go AS, Hylek EM, Phillips KA, et al. Prevalence of diagnosed atrial fibrillation in adults: national implications for rhythm management and stroke prevention: the anticoagulation and risk factors in atrial fibrillation (atria) study. JAMA 2001; 285:2370–5.
3. Verma A, Cairns JA, Mitchell LB, et al. 2014 focused update of the Canadian Cardiovascular Society Guidelines for the management of atrial fibrillation. Can J Cardiol 2014;30:1114–30.
4. Camm AJ, Lip GYH, De Caterina R, et al. 2012 focused update of the ESC Guidelines for the management of atrial fibrillation. Eur Heart J 2012;33(21):2719–47.
5. Spyropoulos AC, Douketis JD. How I treat anticoagulated patients undergoing an elective procedure or surgery. Blood 2012;120:2954–62.
6. Tafur AJ, McBane R, Wysokinski WE, et al. Predictors of major bleeding in periprocedural anticoagulation management. J Thromb Haemost 2012;10:261–7.
7. Witt DM, Delate T, Garcia DA, et al. Risk of thromboembolism, recurrent hemorrhage, and death after warfarin therapy interruption for gastrointestinal tract bleeding. Arch Intern Med 2012;172:1484–91.
8. Jaffer AK, Brotman DJ, Bash LD, et al. Variations in perioperative warfarin management: outcomes and practice patterns at nine hospitals. Am J Med 2010; 123:141–50.
9. Douketis JD, Spyropoulos AC, Spencer FA, et al. Perioperative management of antithrombotic therapy: Antithrombotic Therapy and Prevention of Thrombosis, 9th ed: American College of Chest Physicians Evidence-Based Clinical Practice Guidelines. Chest 2012;141:e326S–350.
10. Tafur A, Douketis JD. Perioperative anticoagulant management in patients with atrial fibrillation: practical implications of recent clinical trials. Pol Arch Med Wewn 2015;125(9):666–71. Available at: http://www.pamw.pl/en/issue/article/26307106. Accessed October 11, 2015.
11. Schulman S, Carrier M, Lee AY, et al. Perioperative management of dabigatran: a prospective cohort study. Circulation 2015;132(3):167–73.
12. Narouze S, Benzon HT, Provenzano DA, et al. Interventional spine and pain procedures in patients on antiplatelet and anticoagulant medications: guidelines from the American Society of Regional Anesthesia and Pain Medicine, the European Society of Regional Anaesthesia and Pain Therapy, the American Academy of Pain Medicine, the International Neuromodulation Society, the North American Neuromodulation Society, and the World Institute of Pain. Reg Anesth Pain Med 2015;40(3):182–212. Available at: http://journals.lww.com/rapm/Fulltext/2015/05000/Interventional_Spine_and_Pain_Procedures_in.2.aspx. Accessed September 28, 2015.
13. Garcia D, Alexander JH, Wallentin L, et al. Management and clinical outcomes in patients treated with apixaban vs warfarin undergoing procedures. Blood 2014; 124:3692–8.
14. Healey JS, Eikelboom J, Douketis J, et al. Periprocedural bleeding and thromboembolic events with dabigatran compared with warfarin: results from the randomized evaluation of long-term anticoagulation therapy (RE-LY) randomized trial. Circulation 2012;126:343–8.
15. Sherwood MW, Douketis JD, Patel MR, et al. Outcomes of temporary interruption of rivaroxaban compared with warfarin in patients with nonvalvular atrial

fibrillation: results from the rivaroxaban once daily, oral, direct factor Xa inhibition compared with vitamin K antagonism for prevention of stroke and embolism trial in atrial fibrillation (ROCKET AF). Circulation 2014;129:1850–9.

16. Beyer-Westendorf J, Förster K, Pannach S, et al. Rates, management, and outcome of rivaroxaban bleeding in daily care: results from the Dresden NOAC registry. Blood 2014;124:955–62.

17. Kearon C. A conceptual framework for two phases of anticoagulant treatment of venous thromboembolism. J Thromb Haemost 2012;10:507–11.

18. Decousus H, Leizorovicz A, Parent F, et al. A clinical trial of vena caval filters in the prevention of pulmonary embolism in patients with proximal deep-vein thrombosis. Prévention du Risque d'Embolie Pulmonaire par Interruption Cave Study Group. N Engl J Med 1998;338:409–15.

19. Kearon C, Akl EA, Comerota AJ, et al. Antithrombotic therapy for VTE disease: antithrombotic therapy and prevention of thrombosis, 9th ed: American College of Chest Physicians Evidence-Based Clinical Practice Guidelines. Chest 2012; 141:e419S–94S.

20. Baron TH, Kamath PS, McBane RD. Antithrombotic therapy and invasive procedures. N Engl J Med 2013;369:1077–80.

21. Vanassche T, Lauw MN, Connolly SJ, et al. Heparin bridging in peri-procedural management of new oral anticoagulant: a bridge too far? Eur Heart J 2014;35: 1831–3.

22. Siegal D, Yudin J, Kaatz S, et al. Periprocedural heparin bridging in patients receiving vitamin K antagonists: systematic review and meta-analysis of bleeding and thromboembolic rates. Circulation 2012;126:1630–9.

23. Douketis JD, Healey JS, Brueckmann M, et al. Perioperative bridging anticoagulation during dabigatran or warfarin interruption among patients who had an elective surgery or procedure. Substudy of the RE-LY trial. Thromb Haemost 2015; 113:625–32.

24. Douketis JD, Spyropoulos AC, Kaatz S, et al. Perioperative bridging anticoagulation in patients with atrial fibrillation. N Engl J Med 2015;373:823–33.

25. Spyropoulos AC, Turpie AGG. Perioperative bridging interruption with heparin for the patient receiving long-term anticoagulation. Curr Opin Pulm Med 2005;11: 373–9.

26. Holbrook A, Schulman S, Witt DM, et al. Evidence-based management of anticoagulant therapy: antithrombotic therapy and prevention of thrombosis, 9th ed: American College of Chest Physicians Evidence-Based Clinical Practice Guidelines. Chest 2012;141:e152S–84S.

27. Curtis R, Schweitzer A, van Vlymen J. Reversal of warfarin anticoagulation for urgent surgical procedures. Can J Anaesth 2015;62:634–49.

28. Cuker A, Siegal DM, Crowther MA, et al. Laboratory measurement of the anticoagulant activity of the non-vitamin K oral anticoagulants. J Am Coll Cardiol 2014; 64:1128–39.

29. Siegal DM. Managing target-specific oral anticoagulant associated bleeding including an update on pharmacological reversal agents. J Thromb Thrombolysis 2015;39:395–402.

30. Glund S, Moschetti V, Norris S, et al. A randomised study in healthy volunteers to investigate the safety, tolerability and pharmacokinetics of idarucizumab, a specific antidote to dabigatran. Thromb Haemost 2015;113:943–51.

31. Pollack CV, Reilly PA, Eikelboom J, et al. Idarucizumab for dabigatran reversal. N Engl J Med 2015;373:511–20.

32. Lu G, DeGuzman FR, Hollenbach SJ, et al. A specific antidote for reversal of anti-coagulation by direct and indirect inhibitors of coagulation factor Xa. Nat Med 2013;19:446–51.

33. Curnutte J, Lu G, Barron L, et al. ANNEXA-R: a phase 3 randomized, double-blind, placebo-controlled trial, demonstrating reversal of rivaroxaban-induced anticoagulation in older subjects by adexanet alfa (PRT064445), a universal antidote for factor Xa (FXA) inhibitors. J Am Coll Cardiol 2015;65(10_S).

Reversal Agents for the Direct Oral Anticoagulants

Jack E. Ansell, MD*

KEYWORDS

- Anticoagulants • Direct oral anticoagulants • Antidotes • Reversal agents • Bleeding
- Hemorrhage • Adverse events • Idarucizumab

KEY POINTS

- The new direct oral anticoagulants have a bleeding risk profile better than the vitamin K antagonists, but are still associated with serious bleeding.
- The new direct oral anticoagulants were developed without specific reversal agents.
- Current recommendations for reversal of the new direct oral anticoagulants when major bleeding occurs include the use of prothrombin complex concentrates.
- There are 3 specific reversal agents in development for the direct oral anticoagulants, with one of them, idarucizumab, recently approved for clinical use.

INTRODUCTION

Oral anticoagulants, because of their intended function to impair coagulation and prevent or retard thrombus development, are associated with an almost obligatory incidence of bleeding ranging from nuisance bleeding to life-threatening and fatal bleeding. This bleeding incidence is well documented with the traditional oral anticoagulant, warfarin, one of the vitamin K antagonists (VKAs).[1] This class of drugs is responsible for the most emergency hospitalizations due to an adverse drug event (bleeding),[2] the most emergency room visits due to an adverse drug event,[3] and the most common cause of death associated with an adverse drug event.[4] Bleeding on warfarin is also an important contributor to the overall costs of anticoagulant therapy.[5] Although most bleeding events occur when patients are therapeutically anticoagulated, VKA therapy is further complicated by poor management that allows patients to be over-anticoagulated and put at a higher risk of anticoagulant-related bleeding.[6] Additional factors, such as poorly controlled hypertension and other comorbidities,

Disclosures: Dr J.E. Ansell serves on the Scientific Advisory Board of Perosphere, Inc and has equity interest in Perosphere, Inc. He also reports consultant activities and honoraria from Bristol Myers Squibb, Pfizer, Boehringer Ingelheim, Daiichi Sankyo, and Janssen.
Department of Medicine, Hofstra North Shore-LIJ School of Medicine, 500 Hofstra Blvd, Hempstead, NY 11549, USA
* 15 Waterview Way, Long Branch, NJ 07740.
E-mail address: ansellje@gmail.com

Hematol Oncol Clin N Am 30 (2016) 1085–1098
http://dx.doi.org/10.1016/j.hoc.2016.05.006
0889-8588/16/$ – see front matter © 2016 Elsevier Inc. All rights reserved.
hemonc.theclinics.com

further enhance the risk of bleeding, and better management of these comorbidities could lessen the incidence of bleeding. Given this serious potential side effect, it is only natural that one would like to be able to reverse anticoagulation when necessary, especially in the setting of life-threatening bleeding. However, having a reversal agent is not so simple. Questions arise as to how effective is the reversal, will reversal of anticoagulation impact overall outcome of the bleeding event, will reversal improve overall patient outcome, does the reversal agent have any deleterious side effects of its own, will reversal of anticoagulation place the patient at an undue risk of a thrombotic event, and will the reversal agent be expensive and possibly not cost-effective. Many of these questions are explored in the following discussion because such agents apply to the new direct oral anticoagulants (DOACs) as well as to warfarin.

WHEN WILL REVERSAL AGENTS BE NEEDED?

The decision to use a reversal agent depends on many factors, including its documented or perceived effectiveness, cost, side-effect profile, and the risk of allowing thrombosis to break through when coagulation is corrected. An effective, inexpensive agent with minimal or no side effects would likely be used more often and for lesser degrees of bleeding than an expensive agent, or one that has potential side effects, or one that has questionable value in improving overall outcome. For reversal of warfarin anticoagulation, vitamin K might fit better in the former category, whereas prothrombin complex concentrates would fit better in the latter category. Given the current complexity and cost structure of reversal agents for the VKAs and the DOACs, it is likely that such agents will be used mostly for patients with major, hemodynamically unstable and life-threatening bleeding or bleeding into a vital organ. They could also be indicated for patients requiring emergent surgery or intervention who are currently on an anticoagulant or patients sustaining severe trauma who might be at great risk of life-threatening bleeding, but without detectable bleeding at the moment. Agents might be used in drug overdose and might even be considered to shorten the interval when an anticoagulant needs to be discontinued for an elective procedure in a patient with a strong underlying thrombotic risk.

ATTRIBUTES OF A USEFUL REVERSAL AGENT

In considering the DOACs and potential reversal agents, one would like an agent that is readily available to clinicians on the front lines, that acts rapidly to reverse anticoagulation and produces sustained normalization of coagulation, that has no significant side effects, does not induce a prothrombotic state, allows re-anticoagulation in the short term if needed, does not induce tolerance, and is relatively inexpensive or cost-effective (**Box 1**). It should also have the potential to improve patient outcomes from the bleeding event, but whether the agent actually halts the bleeding or changes the clinical outcome is as much dependent on the source, size, and location of the bleed as it is on the reversal agent. Demonstrating improved outcomes will be difficult, if not impossible, in a randomized fashion when dealing with life-threatening bleeding.

DO THE VITAMIN K ANTAGONISTS HAVE A REVERSAL AGENT?

The VKAs produce their anticoagulant effect by targeting a key enzyme in the vitamin K pathway, vitamin K oxide reductase complex 1, leading to a decrease in normal functioning vitamin K–dependent coagulation factors (factors II, VII, IX, and X and other vitamin K–dependent proteins).[6] As a result, the prothrombin time (PT), expressed as an international normalized ratio (INR), and the activated partial

> **Box 1**
> **Desired attributes of a reversal agent for the direct oral anticoagulants**
>
> - Readily available at the point of care
> - Acts rapidly
> - Produces sustained normalization of coagulation
> - Has no significant side effects
> - Does not induce a prothrombotic state
> - Allows for re-anticoagulation after control of the acute bleeding event
> - Does not induce tolerance and can be used repetitively, if needed, in the short or long term
> - Does not induce an immune response
> - Inexpensive or cost-effective
> - Has the potential to improve patient outcome from the bleeding event

thromboplastin time (aPTT) become prolonged with the INR being most reflective of therapeutic levels of anticoagulation. Reduced vitamin K will restore normal synthesis of the vitamin K–dependent factors.

The VKAs have a reversal agent,[7] vitamin K, that meets many of the qualities noted above for an ideal agent: readily available, produces sustained normalization of coagulation, has no significant side effects (very rare anaphylaxis when administered rapidly), does not induce a prothrombotic state, does not induce tolerance, and is inexpensive. Unfortunately, its major limitation is that it takes 12 to 24 hours to achieve significant normalization of coagulation based on the time it takes for synthesis of the vitamin K–dependent coagulation factors. As such, it is impractical in the setting of major or life-threatening bleeding or need for urgent surgery. There may also be some degree of difficulty in re-anticoagulation depending on the dose of vitamin K used to restore coagulation.

Rapid correction of coagulation requires replacement of the vitamin K–dependent factors, which can be done by administering fresh frozen plasma (FFP) or prothrombin complex concentrates (PCCs), which contain high concentrations of the vitamin K–dependent coagulation factors (II, VII, IX, and X).[7] FFP has several drawbacks, including high-volume infusions and the potential for fluid overload, longer preparation time, febrile and allergic reactions, hemolytic reactions, transmission of infection, and induction of transfusion-associated acute lung injury.[8,9] PCCs are highly concentrated preparations of the vitamin K–dependent coagulation factors and have the advantage of being able to normalize coagulation within minutes of a brief infusion using small volumes of concentrate.[10,11] Until recently, only 3-factor PCCs were available in the United States (containing very limited amounts of factor VII), but 4-factor PCC is now available. Both concentrates have been shown to rapidly correct the INR when compared with FFP, but there is still controversy about the potential to improve overall outcome.[10] Sarode and colleagues[12] recently evaluated the ability of 4-factor PCC compared with FFP to control bleeding and improve outcome in a randomized, open-label trial in 202 patients with warfarin-related bleeding. Although PCC more rapidly corrected the INR compared with FFP (62.2% of the PCC group vs 9.6% of the FFP groups achieved an INR of ≤1.3), overall patient outcomes were not significantly different (effective hemostasis was achieved in 72.4% vs 65.4% [95% confidence interval: −5.8 to 19.9] in the PCC vs FFP groups, respectively). There was no difference in red blood cell transfusion requirements, length of hospital stay, thromboembolic events, or deaths. Not surprisingly, there was a higher incidence of congestive heart failure in the FFP group (12.8%; median volume transfused = 813.5 mL) than in the PCC group (4.5%; median volume infused = 99.4 mL).

The major safety concern of PCCs is their potential for creating a prothrombotic state and inducing thromboembolism.[13,14] Several studies have documented this potential, and in a meta-analysis of 27 studies (1032 patients) of 3- or 4-factor PCCs to reverse VKA-induced coagulopathy (almost all retrospective or prospective cohort studies), Dentali and colleagues[15] found a 0.7% and 1.8% incidence of thromboembolism, respectively. This low rate must be balanced against the benefits of reducing major bleeding, but such proof will be difficult to demonstrate outside of randomized trials, which are difficult to conduct in these high-risk patients.

Regardless of the controversy over the benefit and value of reversal agents for the VKAs, guidelines generally recommend the administration of vitamin K and 4-factor PCCs to rapidly correct the coagulopathy as measured by the INR in the setting of major bleeding (**Table 1**).[6,7,11,16]

CURRENT STATE OF REVERSAL OF DIRECT ORAL ANTICOAGULANTS BEFORE THE ADVENT OF SPECIFIC AGENTS

In the last 2 decades, research on *oral* anticoagulants has focused predominantly on direct neutralization of 2 specific coagulation factors in the final pathway of coagulation: thrombin (fIIa or activated prothrombin) and fXa (activated factor X). Although ximelagatran (a direct thrombin inhibitor) was the first marketed product of this research, it experienced only a brief lifespan on the European market and was shelved because of hepatic toxicity.[17] Subsequently, 4 new target-specific, direct, oral anticoagulants have been developed, tested, and introduced to the market since 2009: dabigatran etexilate (factor IIa inhibitor), rivaroxaban, apixaban, and edoxaban (all factor

Table 1
Treatments available for reversal of vitamin K antagonist–associated coagulopathy

Parameters	Vitamin K	Fresh Frozen Plasma	3-Factor PCC	4-Factor PCC
Constituents	Vitamin K	Vitamin K–dependent clotting factors	Factors II, IX, X and proteins C and S	Factors II, VII, IX, X and proteins C and S
Administration	Orally or IV	IV	IV	IV
Dose	5–10 mg	10–15 mL/kg	25–50 IU/kg	25–50 IU/kg
Onset of effect	6–8 h	Duration of infusion	15–30 min	15–30 min
Adverse effects	Rare anaphylaxis	Fluid overload; febrile and allergic reactions; viral transmission; transfusion-related acute lung injury	Thromboembolic complications	Thromboembolic complications
Cost	Minimal	Moderate	High	High

Adapted from Quinlan DJ, Eikelboom JW, Weitz JI. Four-factor prothrombin complex concentrate for urgent reversal of vitamin K antagonists in patients with major bleeding. Circulation 2013;128:1180.

Xa inhibitors).[18] They were first shown to be effective in the primary prevention of venous thromboembolism in patients undergoing major orthopedic surgery and are approved for this indication in various countries, but their major indications are for stroke prevention in atrial fibrillation and the initial treatment of acute venous thromboembolism as well as the extended treatment of venous thromboembolism with some agents. Because these agents have a rapid onset and offset of action, a predictable dose effect, minimal drug-drug interaction or dietary interaction, they were developed without the need for monitoring or a specific reversal agent. Although they are shown to have an overall better bleeding risk profile than the VKAs, they are still associated with a clinically significant incidence of major bleeding.[19] Their major advantage in reducing bleeding is related to a consistent reduction in intracranial hemorrhage compared with the VKAs. As a result, they are associated with a reduced rate of fatal bleeding, but site-specific fatal bleeding is not significantly different compared with the VKAs.[20]

There is suggestive evidence that DOAC-related major bleeding, even without a reversal agent, results in outcomes no different than those seen with warfarin-related major bleeding where reversal agents are available. Majeed and colleagues,[21] in an analysis of major bleeding from 5 phase 3 trials of dabigatran, showed that outcome was no different in patients who bled on warfarin versus those on dabigatran, where warfarin has a reversal agent and dabigatran does not. Similar results were seen by Piccini and colleagues,[22] who analyzed results from the ROCKET-AF trial of patients who experienced bleeding on warfarin versus rivaroxaban.

Managing patients with DOAC-associated bleeding requires discontinuation of the anticoagulant, efforts to control bleeding if the site is known, administration of general volume support, red blood cell transfusions as needed, and platelet transfusions if platelet dysfunction or thrombocytopenia is present.[23–26] For patients with recent drug ingestion, gastric lavage with activated charcoal is recommended (within 2–3 hours). Dabigatran, because of its lower protein binding, is amenable to hemodialysis (about 50%–60% of the drug can be removed), whereas the fXa inhibitors are not. For minor or moderate bleeding, these measures are adequate, but for life-threatening bleeding, it is currently advised to administer a prohemostatic agent such as PCCs.[23–27] This recommendation is not based on robust clinical trials, but on evidence acquired from animal studies, reversal of drug activity in healthy individuals, and anecdotal case reports.[28–36] These studies often produce conflicting results because of different animal models, different prohemostatic agents, and most importantly, different coagulation assays used to measure impaired coagulation. In healthy individuals, Eerenberg and colleagues[32] showed that nonactivated 4-factor PCCs reversed the elevated PT and low endogenous thrombin potential induced by rivaroxaban, but it was ineffective in correcting the elevated thrombin time or ecarin clotting time induced by dabigatran. Marlu and colleagues[33] showed that activated PCC (factor eight inhibitor bypass activity) best corrected several rivaroxaban-induced coagulation assays, while others have shown that PCCs can correct dabigatran-induced bleeding in animal models[30,36] and may be effective in real life bleeding.[37]

A recent study did show that PCCs can reduce active bleeding induced by the fXa inhibitor edoxaban. Zahir and colleagues[38] performed punch biopsies in human volunteer subjects and assessed the ability of 4-factor PCC to reduce bleeding. Subjects were pretreated with a 60-mg dose of edoxaban before escalating doses of 4-factor PCC were administered. A dose of 50 IU/kg of PCC reversed the duration of bleeding and endogenous thrombin potential in all subjects, but there was a nonsignificant trend in reduction in bleeding volume.

In summary, DOAC-associated major bleeding can be managed with supportive care, fluid resuscitation, red blood cell transfusions, and, if life-threatening, 4-factor prothrombin concentrates (activated or nonactivated). Current recommendations for the management of bleeding in patients on DOACs are summarized in **Table 2**.

SPECIFIC REVERSAL AGENTS FOR THE DIRECT ORAL ANTICOAGULANTS

Three compounds are currently in development to address the need for specific reversal agents for the DOACs. Idarucizumab is a hybridized murine monoclonal antibody fragment (Fab) with specific activity targeted against dabigatran. It was recently approved by the US Food and Drug Administration (FDA) for clinical use.[39] Andexanet alfa is a modified catalytically inactive recombinant human factor Xa with binding specificity for direct and indirect Xa inhibitors. Ciraparantag is a small molecule that binds to the direct and indirect fXa inhibitors as well as dabigatran, removing them from their respective targets and restoring hemostasis.

Idarucizumab: Reversal of the Oral IIa Inhibitor, Dabigatran

Boehringer Ingelheim, the manufacturer of dabigatran, has developed a humanized mouse monoclonal Fab that is targeted specifically to dabigatran.[40] It has similarities to the binding of thrombin to dabigatran, but the antibody has an affinity for dabigatran that is ~350 times stronger than dabigatran's affinity for thrombin. Idarucizumab was shown to reverse the activity of dabigatran (220 mg twice a day × 3 days) as measured by the thrombin time, dilute thrombin time, and other assays[41] shortly after an infusion in a phase 1 trial of 145 healthy volunteers. The drug was well tolerated with minor drug-related effects. Pollack and colleagues[42] reported the interim results of a phase 3 prospective cohort study of idarucizumab's ability to reverse impaired coagulation in 2 groups of patients: 51 who presented with major bleeding and 39 who required urgent surgery (RE-VERSE AD; NCT02104947). Greater than 90% of the patients required anticoagulation for stroke prevention in atrial fibrillation. The median time from the last dose of dabigatran was between 15 and 16 hours for the 2 groups and approximately 75% had an elevated dilute thrombin time at baseline, whereas approximately 90% had an elevated ecarin clotting time (a more sensitive assay for dabigatran). In patients with major bleeding, 35% had intracranial hemorrhage and 39% had gastrointestinal bleeding. The top 5 surgical interventions were bone fractures,[8] acute cholecystitis,[5] catheter placement in acute renal failure,[4] acute appendicitis,[3] and joint/wound infection.[3] Idarucizumab was given in 2 sequential intravenous (IV)

Table 2
Current consensus recommendations for reversal of the target-specific oral anticoagulants

Intervention	Apixaban	Rivaroxaban	Edoxaban	Dabigatran
Oral activated charcoal	Yes	Yes	Yes	Yes
Hemodialysis	No	No	No	Yes
Hemoperfusion with activated charcoal	Possible	Possible	?	Yes
FFP	No	No	No	No
Activated recombinant FVIIa	Unclear	Unclear	Unclear	Unclear
3-Factor PCC	Unclear	Unclear	Unclear	Unclear
4-Factor PCC	Possible	Possible		Possible

Abbreviation: ?, unknown.
Adapted from Kaatz S, Kouides PA, Garcia DA, et al. Guidance on the emergent reversal of oral thrombin and factor Xa inhibitors. Am J Hematol 2012;87:4; with permission.

injections of 2.5 g each. Because of normal dilute thrombin times at baseline, correction of tests could only be determined in 40 patients in the bleeding group and 28 in the surgical group. For the ecarin clotting time, the numbers were 47 and 34, respectively. The dilute thrombin time was normalized in 98% of patients with bleeding and 93% in patients requiring surgery within minutes, and test results remained normal for the subsequent 24 hours (**Fig. 1**). The numbers for the ecarin clotting time were 89% and 88%, respectively. Among 36 patients who underwent a procedure, intraoperative hemostasis was reported to be normal in 33 and only mildly or moderately impaired in 3. Of 35 patients with major bleeding, hemostasis was restored at a median of 11.4 hours. There were 9 deaths in each study group, including 5 fatal bleeding events. There were also 5 patients with thrombotic events (1 patient < 72 hours after idarucizumab given).

In October 2015, idarucizumab (Praxbind) was given FDA approval with indications for the reversal of dabigatran in patients requiring emergency surgery/urgent procedures or in life-threatening or uncontrolled bleeding.[39,43]

Andexanet Alfa: Reversal of the Xa Inhibitors, Rivaroxaban, Apixaban, Edoxaban

Andexanet alfa is a reversal agent developed by Portola Pharmaceuticals for reversal of the direct oral fXa inhibitors. It also has reversal activity for the indirect fXa inhibitor, enoxaparin.[44] Andexanet is a recombinant human factor Xa protein[45] that is modified by elimination of the gla residues and inactivation of its catalytic site by amino acid substitution. Because of this modification, it has no coagulant activity, but it retains its ability to bind factor Xa inhibitors, removing them from their intended target. Andexanet reverses abnormal coagulation assays induced by rivaroxaban or apixaban as shown in preclinical studies and reduces bleeding in animal models.[46] Results of a phase 3 trial were recently published following successful phase 2 studies.[47]

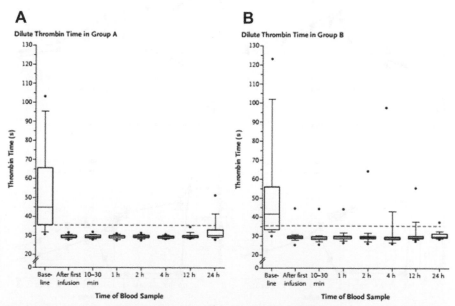

Fig. 1. (*A*) Fifty-one patients with serious bleeding; (*B*) 39 patients who required urgent surgery/intervention. *Filled circles* represent outliers who did not correct clotting times after idarucizumab. (*From* Pollack CV, Reilly PA, Eikelboom J, et al. Idarucizumab for dabigatran reversal. N Engl J Med 2015;373:516; with permission.)

Andexanet was well tolerated in all trials with no serious side effects. In phase 2 trials, investigators found that a continuous infusion of andexanet was required in order to achieve sustained reversal of the fXa inhibitor.[48] Phase 2 studies also showed that tissue factor pathway inhibitor, which binds to andexanet, was lowered following treatment. This latter finding raises concern about creating a prothrombotic state, but to date, no thrombotic episodes have occurred in study subjects, albeit all subjects have been healthy volunteers. In their recent phase 3 report,[47] investigators treated healthy elderly volunteers with either rivaroxaban or apixaban using a bolus injection or bolus followed by a 2-hour infusion of andexanet. In the apixaban and rivaroxaban arms of the study, antifactor Xa activity was reduced by 94% and 92%, respectively, in the treatment arms versus 21% and 18% in the placebo arms, respectively (**Fig. 2**). Differences from placebo were highly significant in each group ($P<.001$). Thrombin generation was also restored in 100% and 96% of the active treatment arms versus 11% and 7% in the placebo arms ($P<.001$ for each drug vs placebo). These changes occurred within minutes after infusion and were sustained for the duration of the infusion in those given a bolus and infusion (see **Fig. 2**). Andexanet was well tolerated by recipients with no serious adverse events. D-dimer and prothrombin fragments 1 and

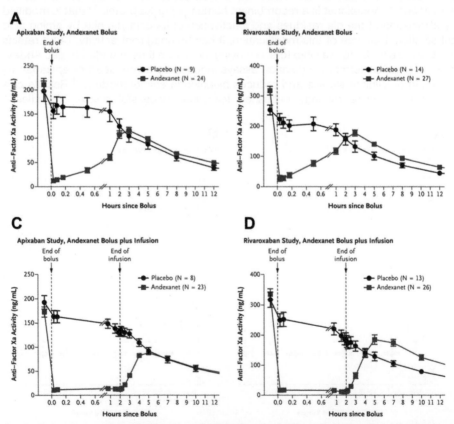

Fig. 2. Time course of antifactor Xa activity before and after administration of a bolus or bolus + infusion of andexanet alfa in healthy elderly volunteers treated with apixaban or rivaroxaban. (*From* Pollack CV, Reilly PA, Eikelboom J, et al. Idarucizumab for dabigatran reversal. N Engl J Med 2015;373:2417; with permission.)

2 were mildly elevated in most subjects and returned to baseline within 24 to 72 hours. Measurements of TFPI were not reported. Nonneutralizing antibodies were detected in 17% versus 2% of drug-treated versus placebo patients. Antibody titers were generally low (except one patient with a titer of 1:2560) and appeared 15 to 30 days after treatment.

This study shows what seems to be effective reversal of apixaban and rivaroxaban in healthy subjects. The drug must be given as a continuous infusion for sustained reversal of anti-fXa activity. The mild prothrombotic profile as measured by select biomarkers maintains the concern as to whether andexanet could precipitate thrombotic events in patients who already are predisposed by having an underlying thrombotic condition. The immune response, although mild, also raises concern as to whether andexanet can be effective in the same patient who might require reversal at some future time.

Ciraparantag: Reversal of Both IIa and Xa Inhibitors

Perosphere, Inc is the developer of ciraparantag (originally PER977), a small synthetic water-soluble compound (512 Da) that was originally synthesized as an agent to bind to, and neutralize, unfractionated and low-molecular-weight heparin.[49] Studies show that ciraparantag noncovalently binds to heparin, enoxaparin, dabigatran, apixaban, rivaroxaban, and edoxaban, preventing the binding of these anticoagulants to their endogenous targets, thereby reversing the anticoagulation induced by these drugs.

Ciraparantag is stable as lyophilized powder (>1 year), has no demonstrable toxic effects in animals, does not affect CYP metabolism, and does not bind to a wide range of cardiovascular drugs.[50] Preclinical studies show that a single IV dose restores normal hemostasis in external (rat tail transection) and internal (liver laceration) bleeding models and corrects abnormal coagulation assays.[51,52]

In a first-in-human trial, 180 healthy volunteers received escalating doses of ciraparantag after receiving a 60-mg dose of edoxaban. An immediate correction of whole blood clotting time was achieved in a dose-response manner with 100 mg being the threshold dose for complete reversal, which was sustained over the next 24 hours without further treatment (**Fig. 3**).[53] The drug was well tolerated with minimal side effects, and there was no evidence of a prothrombotic effect as seen by sequential measurement over 24 hours of prothrombin fragment 1.2, D-dimer, and tissue factor pathway inhibitor. Investigators recently reported that ciraparantag also reverses steady-state dosing of edoxaban and allows for re-anticoagulation with edoxaban within 24 hours, which can once again be reversed with ciraparantag, indicating that tachyphylaxis or resistance to ciraparantag does not develop (see **Fig. 3B, C**).[54] Investigators have also reported on the ability of ciraparantag to reverse the indirect parenteral Xa inhibitor, enoxaparin.[55]

One challenge facing ciraparantag is measuring its effectiveness with standard coagulation assays. Ciraparantag binds to the reagents used for anticoagulating blood in vitro (Na citrate, EDTA, heparin) as well as activating agents used in some tests (celite, kaolin). Because of the molar excess of these agents, the reversal agent is removed from its respective target in vitro, allowing anticoagulation to reassert itself (to varying degrees), and thus, yield false coagulation assays (PT, aPTT, anti-factor Xa). The whole-blood clotting time performed in glass tubes without activating reagents has been shown not only to reflect anticoagulation with the heparin and DOAC anticoagulants but also to show correction following treatment with ciraparantag.[55] Because this is a manual assay and subject to intersubject imprecision, it is not suitable for clinical use. The development of point-of-care automated methods for the whole blood clotting time may resolve this challenge.

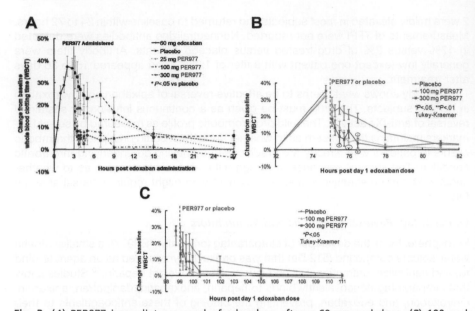

Fig. 3. (*A*) PER977 immediate reversal of edoxaban after a 60-mg oral dose. (*B*) 100 and 300 mg PER977 achieved complete and sustained reversal of steady-state edoxaban on day 3. (*C*) Patients re-anticoagulated with edoxaban on day 4 and reversed with 100 or 300 mg PER977. (*From [A]* Ansell JE, Bakhru S, Laulicht BE, et al. Use of PER977 to reverse the anticoagulant effect of edoxaban. N Engl J Med 2014;339:2142, with permission; and *Data from [C]* Bakhru S, Laulicht B, Jiang X, et al. PER977: a synthetic small molecule which reverses over-dosage and bleeding by the new oral anticoagulants. [abstract]. Circulation 2013;128:A18809; and *From* Steiner S, Bakhru S, Laulicht BE, et al. PER977 (Ciraparantag) reverses edoxaban anticoagulation at steady-state and has no effect on re-anticoagulation at the next scheduled dose. Presented at European Society of Cardiology. London, September 1, 2015; with permission.)

THE FUTURE OF DIRECT ORAL ANTICOAGULANTS REVERSAL AGENTS

Despite the debate as to whether DOAC reversal agents are needed,[56,57] the current agents under development are likely to gain market entry depending on the results of phase 3 trials. Their use, along with the recently approved dabigatran reversal agent, will depend on many factors, including their effectiveness, side-effect profile, and cost. Perhaps the most important consequence as a result of their development will be an increase in the prescription of DOACs and an increase in the treatment of conditions such as atrial fibrillation.[58]

REFERENCES

1. Schulman S, Beyth RJ, Kearon C, et al. Hemorrhagic complications of anticoagulant and thrombolytic treatment. Chest 2008;133:257S–98S.
2. Budnitz DS, Lovegrove MC, Shehab N, et al. Emergency hospitalizations for adverse drug events in older Americans. N Engl J Med 2011;365:2002–12.
3. Budnitz DS, Shehab N, Kegler SR, et al. Medication use leading to emergency department visits for adverse drug events in older adults. Ann Intern Med 2007;147:755–65.

4. Shepherd G, Mohorn P, Yacoub K, et al. Adverse drug reaction deaths reported in United States Vital Statistics, 1999-2006. Ann Pharmacother 2012;46:169–75.
5. Ghate SR, Biskupiak J, Ye X, et al. All-cause bleeding-related health care costs in warfarin-treated patients with atrial fibrillation. J Manag Care Pharm 2011;17: 672–84.
6. Ansell J, Hirsh J, Hylek E, et al. The pharmacology and management of the vitamin K antagonists: ACCP evidence-based clinical practice guidelines. Chest 2008;133:160S–98S.
7. Garcia DA, Crowther MA. Reversal of warfarin: case-based practice recommendations. Circulation 2012;125:2944–7.
8. Pandey S, Vyas GN. Adverse effects of plasma transfusion. Transfusion 2012; 52(Suppl 1):65S–79S.
9. Sokolovic M, Pastores SM. Transfusion therapy and acute lung injury. Expert Rev Respir Med 2010;4:387–93.
10. Khorsand N, Kooistra HAM, van Hest RM, et al. A systematic review of prothrombin complex concentrate dosing strategies to reverse vitamin K antagonist therapy. Thromb Res 2014;135:9–19.
11. Holbrook A, Schulman S, Witt DM, et al. Evidence-based management of anticoagulant therapy: antithrombotic therapy and prevention of thrombosis, 9th ed: American College of Chest Physicians evidence-based clinical practice guidelines. Chest 2012;141(2 Suppl):e152S–84S.
12. Sarode R, Milling TJ, Refaai MA, et al. Efficacy and safety of a four-factor prothrombin complex concentrate (4F-PCC) in patients on Vitamin K antagonists presenting with major bleeding: a randomized, plasma-controlled, phase IIIb study. Circulation 2013;128:1234–43.
13. Grottke O, Braunschweig T, Spronk HMH, et al. Increasing concentrations of prothrombin complex concentrate induce DIC in a pig model of coagulopathy with blunt liver injury. Blood 2011;118:1943–51.
14. Dusel CH, Grundmann C, Eich S, et al. Identification of prothrombin as a major thrombogenic agent in prothrombin complex concentrates. Blood Coagul Fibrinolysis 2004;15:405–11.
15. Dentali F, Marches C, Pierfranceschi MG, et al. Safety of prothrombin complex concentrates for rapid anticoagulation reversal of vitamin K antagonists. Thromb Haemost 2011;106:429–38.
16. Quinlan DJ, Eikelboom JW, Weitz JI. Four-factor prothrombin complex concentrate for urgent reversal of vitamin K antagonists in patients with major bleeding. Circulation 2013;128:1179–81.
17. Available at: http://www.medscape.com/viewarticle/788220. Accessed December 8, 2015.
18. Weitz JI, Eikelboom JW, Samama MM. New antithrombotic drugs: antithrombotic therapy and prevention of thrombosis, 9th ed: American College of Chest Physicians evidence-based clinical practice guidelines. Chest 2012;141(2 Suppl): e120S–51S.
19. Chai-Adisaksopha C, Crowther M, Isayama T, et al. The impact of bleeding complications in patients receiving target-specific oral anticoagulants: a systematic review and meta-analysis. Blood 2014;124:2450–8.
20. Skaistis J, Tagami T. Risk of fatal bleeding in episodes of major bleeding with new oral anticoagulants and vitamin K antagonists: a systematic review and meta-analysis. PLoS One 2015;10(9):e0137444.

21. Majeed A, Hwang HG, Connolly SJ, et al. Management and outcomes of major bleeding during treatment with dabigatran or warfarin. Circulation 2013;128: 2325–32.
22. Piccini JP, Garg J, Patel MR, et al. Management of major bleeding events in patients treated with rivaroxaban vs. warfarin: results from the ROCKET AF trial. Eur Heart J 2014;35:1873–80.
23. Siegal DM. Managing target-specific oral anticoagulant associated bleeding including an update on pharmacological reversal agents. J Thromb Thrombolysis 2015;39:395–402.
24. Jackson LR, Becker RC. Novel oral anticoagulants: pharmacology, coagulation measures, and considerations for reversal. J Thromb Thrombolysis 2014;37: 380–91.
25. Kaatz S, Kouides PA, Garcia DA, et al. Guidance on the emergent reversal of oral thrombin and factor Xa inhibitors. Am J Hematol 2012;87:S141–5.
26. Miesbach W, Seifried E. New direct oral anticoagulants-current therapeutic options and treatment recommendations for bleeding complications. Thromb Haemost 2012;108:625–32.
27. Miller MP, Trujillo TC, Nordenholz KE. Practical considerations in emergency management of bleeding in the setting of target-specific oral anticoagulants. Am J Emerg Med 2014;32:375–82.
28. Perzhorn E, Gruber A, Tinel H, et al. Reversal of rivaroxaban anticoagulation by haemostatic agents in rats and primates. Thromb Haemost 2013;110:162–72.
29. Lambourne MD, Eltringham-Smith LJ, Gataiance S, et al. Prothrombin complex concentrates reduce blood loss in murine coagulopathy induced by warfarin, but not in that induced by dabigatran etexilate. J Thromb Haemost 2012;10: 1830–40.
30. Pragst I, Zeitler SH, Doerr B, et al. Reversal of dabigatran anticoagulation by prothrombin complex concentrate (Beriplex P/N) in a rabbit model. J Thromb Haemost 2012;10:1841–8.
31. Dinkelaar J, Molenaar PJ, Ninivaggi M, et al. In vitro assessment, using thrombin generation, of the applicability of prothrombin complex concentrate as an antidote for rivaroxaban. J Thromb Haemost 2013;11:1111–8.
32. Eerenberg ES, Kamphuisen PW, Sijpkens MK, et al. Reversal of rivaroxaban and dabigatran by prothrombin complex concentrate. A randomized, placebo-controlled, crossover study in healthy subjects. Circulation 2011;124:1573–9.
33. Marlu R, Hodaj E, Paris A, et al. Effect of non-specific reversal agents on anticoagulant activity of dabigatran and rivaroxaban. Thromb Haemost 2012;108: 217–24.
34. Fukuda T, Honda Y, Kamisato C, et al. Reversal of anticoagulant effects of edoxaban, an oral, direct factor Xa inhibitor, with haemostatic agents. Thromb Haemost 2012;107:253–9.
35. Dickneite G, Hoffman M. Reversing the new oral anticoagulants with prothrombin complex concentrates (PCCs): what is the evidence? Thromb Haemost 2014;111: 189–98.
36. Honickel M, Braunschweig T, van Ryn J, et al. Prothrombin complex concentrate is effective in treating the anticoagulant effects of dabigatran in a porcine polytrauma model. Anesthesiology 2015;123:1350–61.
37. Diaz MQ, Borobia AM, Nunez MAR, et al. Use of prothrombin complex concentrates for urgent reversal of dabigatran in the emergency department. Haematologica 2013;98:e143–4.

38. Zahir H, Brown KS, Vandell A, et al. Edoxaban effects on bleeding following punch biopsy and reversal by a 4-factor prothrombin complex concentrate. Circulation 2014;131:82–90.
39. Available at: http://www.fda.gov/NewsEvents/Newsroom/PressAnnouncements/ucm467300.htm. Accessed December 8, 2015.
40. Schiele F, van Ryn J, Canada K, et al. A specific antidote for dabigatran: functional and structural characterization. Blood 2013;121:3554–62.
41. Glund S, Stangier J, Schmohl M, et al. A specific antidote for dabigatran: immediate, complete and sustained reversal of dabigatran induced anticoagulation in healthy male volunteers. Circulation 2013;128:A17765.
42. Pollack CV, Reilly PA, Eikelboom J, et al. Idarucizumab for dabigatran reversal. N Engl J Med 2015;373:511–20.
43. Available at: http://www.accessdata.fda.gov/drugsatfda_docs/label/2015/761025lbl.pdf. Accessed December 8, 2015.
44. Crowther M, Lu G, Conley P, et al. Reversal of factor Xa inhibitors-induced anticoagulation in healthy subjects by andexanet alfa. Crit Care Med 2014;42:pA1469.
45. Lu G, DeGuzman FR, Hollenbach SJ, et al. A specific antidote for reversal of anticoagulation by direct and indirect inhibitors of coagulation factor Xa. Nat Med 2013;19:446–51.
46. Shah N, Rattu MA. Reversal agents for anticoagulants: focus on andexanet alfa. Am Student Res J 2014;1:16–28.
47. Siegal DM, Curnutte JT, Connolly SJ, et al. Andexanet alfa for the reversal of factor Xa inhibitor activity. N Engl J Med 2015;373(25):2413–24.
48. Crowther M, Vandana M, Michael K, et al. A phase 2 randomized, double-blind, placebo-controlled trial demonstrating reversal of rivaroxaban-induced anticoagulation in healthy subjects by andexanet alfa, an antidote for FXa inhibitors [abstract]. Blood 2013;122:3636.
49. Laulicht B, Bakhru S, Jiang X, et al. Antidote for new oral anticoagulants: mechanism of action and binding specificity of PER977. [abstract]. Presented at the 24th Congress of the International Society on Thrombosis and Haemostasis. Amsterdam, June 29–July 4, 2013. Available at: http://www.eventure-online.com/eventure/publicAbstractView.do?id=226718&congressId=6839.
50. Laulicht B, Bakhru S, Lee C, et al. Small molecule antidote for anticoagulants. Circulation 2012;126(21) [abstract 11395].
51. Bakhru S, Laulicht B, Jiang X, et al. PER977: a synthetic small molecule which reverses over-dosage and bleeding by the new oral anticoagulants [abstract]. Circulation 2013;128:A18809.
52. Bakhru S, Laulicht B, Jiang X, et al. Reversal of anticoagulant-induced bleeding in external and internal bleeding models by PER977, a small molecule anticoagulant antidote [abstract]. Circulation 2014;130:A19361.
53. Ansell JE, Bakhru S, Laulicht BE, et al. Use of PER977 to reverse the anticoagulant effect of edoxaban. N Engl J Med 2014;339:2141–2.
54. Steiner S, Bakhru S, Laulicht BE, Costin J. PER977 (Ciraparantag) reverses edoxaban anticoagulation at steady-state and has no effect on re-anticoagulation at the next scheduled dose. Presented at European Society of Cardiology. London, September 1, 2015.
55. Costin J, Laulicht B, Bakhru S, et al. PER977 reverses low molecular weight heparin in addition to IIa and Xa new oral anticoagulants [abstract]. J Am Coll Cardiol 2015;65(10 Suppl). http://dx.doi.org/10.1016/S0735-1097/(15)62056-3.

56. Roldan V, Marin F. Pro antidote for new anticoagulants—specific target of inhibition requires a specific target for neutralization. Thromb Haemost 2012;108:621–2.
57. Eerenberg ES, Levi M, Buller HR. Contra: antidotes for novel anticoagulants—do we really need them. Thromb Haemost 2012;108:623–4.
58. Sarich TC, Seltzer JH, Berkowitz SD, et al. Novel oral anticoagulants and reversal agents: considerations for clinical development. Am Heart J 2015;169:751–7.

The Intrinsic Pathway of Coagulation as a Target for Antithrombotic Therapy

Allison P. Wheeler, MD, MSCI[a,b,]*, David Gailani, MD[a,c]

KEYWORDS

- Intrinsic pathway • Contact activation • Thrombosis • Factor XI • Factor XII

KEY POINTS

- The term intrinsic pathway refers to a series of sequential reactions involving the plasma proteins factors VIII, IX, XI, and XII; prekallikrein; and high-molecular-weight kininogen, which are required for initiation of coagulation in the activated partial thromboplastin time assay.
- Certain components of the intrinsic pathway that serve a limited role in hemostasis (factor XI), or are not required for hemostasis (factor XII, prekallikrein, and high-molecular-weight kininogen), are required for clot formation in animal models of thrombosis.
- Epidemiologic data indicate that factor XI contributes to venous thromboembolism and ischemic stroke, and may contribute to myocardial infarction in humans, whereas factor XII likely contributes to thrombus formation when blood is exposed to artificial surfaces, such as during cardiopulmonary bypass and extracorporeal membrane oxygenation.
- Reducing factor XI level to 20% of normal by antisense oligonucleotide technology was more effective than standard-dose low-molecular-weight heparin in preventing venous thrombosis during knee replacement surgery, without comprising intraoperative or postoperative hemostasis.
- By targeting components of the intrinsic pathway of coagulation with therapeutic inhibitors, it may be possible to uncouple antithrombotic effects from anticoagulant (antihemostatic) effects, improving the safety of antithrombotic therapy.

Disclosure: A.P. Wheeler has received consultants fees from Bayer Pharmaceuticals and Novo Nordisk; D. Gailani has received consultants fees and research support from Aronora, Bayer Pharmaceuticals, Bristol-Myers Squibb, Dyax Corp., Instrument Laboratory, Ionis, Novartis, and Ono Pharmaceuticals.
Funding: NIH (HL58837; HL81326).
a Department of Pathology, Microbiology and Immunology, Vanderbilt University, C-3321A Medical Center North, 1161 21st Avenue, Nashville, TN 37232, USA; b Department of Pediatrics, Vanderbilt University, 397 Preston Research Building, 2220 Pierce Ave, Nashville, TN 37232, USA; c Hematology/Oncology Division, Department of Medicine, Vanderbilt University, 777 Preston Research Building, 2220 Pierce Avenue, Nashville, TN 37232, USA
* Corresponding author. Department of Pathology, Immunology and Microbiology, Vanderbilt University, C-2213A Medical Center North, 1161 21st Avenue, Nashville, TN 37232-2561.
E-mail address: allison.p.wheeler@vanderbilt.edu

Hematol Oncol Clin N Am 30 (2016) 1099–1114
http://dx.doi.org/10.1016/j.hoc.2016.05.007
0889-8588/16/© 2016 Elsevier Inc. All rights reserved.

INTRODUCTION

The protease thrombin makes essential contributions to hemostasis through its capacity to catalyze conversion of fibrinogen to fibrin, to stimulate platelet and vascular endothelial cells, and to activate plasma coagulation factors.[1] Thrombin also plays a central role in thrombosis, and several approaches have been developed to manipulate this enzyme to achieve an antithrombotic effect. The activity of thrombin or factor (f) Xa (the enzyme responsible for converting prothrombin to thrombin) can be inhibited directly with drugs targeting the enzyme active sites (argatroban, dabigatran, and bivalirudin for thrombin; rivaroxaban, apixaban, and edoxaban for fXa),[2] or indirectly with heparin-related compounds (unfractionated or low-molecular-weight heparin or fondaparinux) that enhance the activity of the plasma inhibitor antithrombin.[3] Alternatively, synthesis of prothrombin and fX, the precursors of thrombin and fXa, can be reduced with vitamin K antagonists such as warfarin.[4] Use of these effective antithrombotic strategies comes with a well-recognized cost. Thrombin and fXa serve vital roles in hemostasis, and therapies directed at them increase bleeding. Use of heparin is associated with major bleeding rates of up to 3%, and 2% to 13% with warfarin.[3–5] Newer oral thrombin and fXa inhibitors seem to cause less bleeding than the older drugs, and are easier to use.[2,6] However, because of their mechanisms of action, there are limits on the types of patients who are eligible to receive them, the clinical settings in which they can be used, and the intensity of anticoagulation that can be applied.

The strategy of targeting thrombin and/or fXa to achieve an antithrombotic effect is based on the intuitive notion that formation of an intravascular thrombus is largely the result of dysregulation of processes normally involved in hemostasis. This premise is currently being reconsidered. There is substantial interest in developing and testing novel therapies that target the proteases of the plasma intrinsic pathway of coagulation (fIX, fXI, fXII, and prekallikrein [PK]) for treating or preventing thromboembolic disorders.[7–9] The physiologic importance of the intrinsic pathway has been questioned since the original descriptions of the cascade-waterfall model of coagulation[10,11] because, although some components of the pathway are clearly required for hemostasis, others are not.[12] This article reviews preclinical and clinical data supporting the hypothesis that components of the intrinsic pathway, and perhaps the intrinsic pathway itself, contribute to thrombosis, and that a useful antithrombotic effect can be achieved by targeting plasma factors that serve minor roles in hemostasis. To understand how the intrinsic pathway might contribute to thrombosis, we first need to review how understanding of this pathway has evolved over the past 50 years.

THE INTRINSIC PATHWAY IN MODELS OF BLOOD COAGULATION
The Cascade-Waterfall Model of Thrombin Generation

The cascade-waterfall hypotheses of intrinsic coagulation was first proposed in 2 landmark articles in 1964 by Macfarlane,[10] and by Davie and Ratnoff.[11] In subsequent models based on this scheme, the process of thrombin generation is the result of amplification of a procoagulant signal initiated by conversion of fXII to fXIIa, followed sequentially by activation of the enzyme precursors fXI, fIX, fX, and prothrombin (**Fig. 1**A). At the time this model was proposed, it was recognized that much of the cascade could be bypassed through a process involving fVIIa (see **Fig. 1**A),[10,11] but the importance of this was not clear. The scheme in **Fig. 1**A depicts the major enzyme reactions that contribute to plasma clotting in the activated partial thromboplastin time (aPTT) and prothrombin time (PT) assays used in clinical practice. There are 2 triggering mechanisms that converge at the level of fX activation. Activation through the intrinsic pathway (see **Fig. 1**A, yellow arrows) is assessed by the aPTT assay, and is initiated by a process involving fXII called contact activation (discussed later). In the PT assay, coagulation is triggered through the extrinsic pathway by adding tissue extracts to the plasma that contain tissue factor (TF),[13] a cofactor for fVIIa.

The sequential steplike nature of the coagulation cascade implies that complete deficiency of any component would break the reaction chain and cause bleeding, but this is not what is observed in clinical practice.[13] Absence of fIX or its cofactor fVIII causes the severe bleeding disorder hemophilia, implying an important role for the intrinsic pathway in hemostasis.[14] However, complete fXII deficiency, despite causing a marked prolongation of the aPTT, does not cause abnormal bleeding,[7,12] whereas fXI deficiency causes a mild hemorrhagic disorder that involves tissues distinct from those commonly affected in fIX or fVIII deficiency.[12,15,16] These observations indicate that the classic intrinsic pathway does not accurately describe the manner in which its components contribute to hemostasis, and have led to revisions in the models that are more in line with clinical phenotypes.

Tissue Factor–initiated Thrombin Generation: The Role of Factor XI

It is the current consensus that thrombin generation at a site of vascular injury is initiated primarily by fVIIa in complex with TF (**Fig. 1**B), an integral membrane protein expressed on cells underlying blood vessel endothelium.[17,18] FVIIa/TF initiates coagulation by activating fX, as in the PT assay (see **Fig. 1**A), and also activates fIX, which sustains fXa and thrombin production. The protease precursors (prothrombin, fVII, fIX, and fX) and cofactors (TF, fVa, and fVIIIa) shown within the gray area in **Fig. 1**B form the core mechanism for thrombin generation in almost all vertebrate organisms.[19] Total deficiency of any one of these proteins results in a severe bleeding disorder or is not compatible with life.[20] This core mechanism is the target of all currently approved anticoagulants. Thus, it is to be expected that use of these compounds will increase bleeding risk.

In addition to the core proteins, mammals have fXI, the precursor of the protease fXIa (see **Fig. 1**B).[21,22] Severe fXI deficiency may cause excessive bleeding with trauma, particularly if tissues with robust fibrinolytic activity, such as the oropharynx or urinary tract, are involved.[12,15,16] However, unlike fIX deficiency, severe spontaneous bleeding is not common in fXI deficiency. Furthermore, bleeding is highly variable, and some fXI-deficient individuals are asymptomatic despite marked abnormalities in the aPTT. Although fXI is activated by fXIIa in the cascade-waterfall model (see **Fig. 1**A), the absence of abnormal bleeding in fXII-deficient individuals indicates that other mechanisms for fXI activation must exist. For example, thrombin generated early in coagulation can activate fXI (see **Fig. 1**B, green arrow).[23–25]

In the scheme shown in **Fig. 1**B, fXIa sustains thrombin generation by activating fIX, rather than contributing to initiation of thrombin formation, as in the cascade-waterfall model and the aPTT assay. A key feature of the newer model is that there are 2 mechanisms for fIX activation, explaining the differences in bleeding phenotypes associated with fIX and fXI deficiencies. In the absence of fXI, fIX still contributes to thrombin production because it can be activated by factor VIIa/TF. Clinical observations suggest that factor VIIa/TF is probably the more important mechanism for fIX activation. Along similar lines, the different phenotypes associated with fXI and fXII deficiency are explained by the presence of more than 1 mechanism for fXI activation. Current models of thrombin generation often do not include a role for fXII, based largely on the observation that fXII deficiency is not associated with a bleeding diathesis. However, as discussed later, it does not necessarily follow that fXIIa does not contribute to thrombin generation under any circumstances.

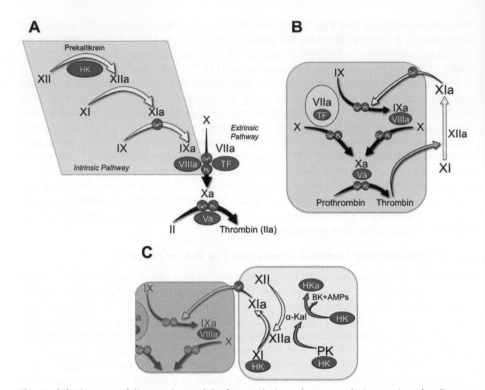

Fig. 1. (*A*) The waterfall/cascade model of coagulation: the proteolytic reactions leading to thrombin generation during plasma coagulation initiated through the intrinsic (*yellow arrows*) and extrinsic (fVIIa/tissue factor [TF]) pathways. The zymogen (precursor) forms of plasma trypsin-like proteases involved in coagulation are represented by the black Roman numerals, and their active protease forms by Roman numerals followed by a lowercase "a." PK is the zymogen of the protease alpha-kallikrein. Protein cofactors are shown in red ovals, and reactions requiring calcium (Ca^{2+}) or phospholipid (PL) are indicated in blue. A feature of this model is that fXa and thrombin formation can be initiated through 2 distinct pathways. In the PT assay, coagulation is initiated by addition of the cofactor TF to plasma. TF in complex with fVIIa forms the extrinsic pathway of coagulation, which activates fX to fXa. In the activated partial thromboplastin time, addition of a negatively charged substance (usually a purified earth) to plasma triggers activation of fXII, and sets off the series of enzymatic reactions referred to as the intrinsic pathway of coagulation. The intrinsic pathway protease fIXa is an activator of fX in this model, bypassing the need for fVIIa/TF. fXa converts prothrombin to the protease thrombin, which then induces coagulation of plasma by converting fibrinogen to fibrin. (*B*) fVIIa/TF-initiated model of coagulation. The model presents the current understanding of the major plasma protease-substrate interactions during thrombin generation in vivo. The nomenclature and symbols are the same as those used in (*A*). Coagulation is initiated by exposure of the fVIIa/TF complex to blood, leading to the activation of fIX and fX. Early in the process, fXa converts prothrombin to thrombin to initiate coagulation, whereas fIXa generates more fXa to sustain the process. In this scheme, fXIa may contribute to thrombin generation by converting additional fIX to fIXa. Because fXII deficiency does not cause a hemostatic abnormality, it is thought that fXI is converted to fXIa by a protease other than fXII. For example, fXI can be activated by thrombin (*green arrow*). In contrast with the cascade/waterfall model in (*A*), here the intrinsic pathway (*yellow arrows*) triggered by initial fVIIa/TF-mediated thrombin generation is not part of mechanism for initiating coagulation, but functions to sustain fIX activation, and ultimately thrombin generation, to maintain the integrity of a clot over time. (*C*) The kallikrein-kinin (contact activation) system. When blood is exposed to a variety of surfaces

The Kallikrein-Kinin System and Contact Activation

The plasma protease precursors fXII and PK and the cofactor high-molecular-weight kininogen (HK) form the plasma kallikrein-kinin system.[26,27] fXII was first identified as a plasma constituent missing in a patient with a very long aPTT, but without abnormal bleeding. Subsequent work identified PK and HK as necessary for normal fXII activation in the aPTT. When plasma is exposed to artificial surfaces or anionic substances, fXII and PK undergo reciprocal conversion to fXIIa and alpha-kallikrein by a process called contact activation (**Fig. 1C**).[12,26,27] HK serves as a cofactor during this process. In the aPTT assay, a purified earth such as silica or Celite is used to induce contact activation, with the resulting fXIIa promoting thrombin generation by activating fXI. The absence of bleeding symptoms in individuals lacking fXII, PK, or HK shows that these proteins are not required for hemostasis,[12] either because they do not normally contribute to thrombin generation or because other mechanisms, such as thrombin-mediated feedback activation of fXI (see **Fig. 1B**), compensate for their absence. The kallikrein-kinin system is thought to contribute to several homeostatic and host-defense mechanisms, including inflammation and the innate immune response to microorganisms.[26–29] It is also clear that fXIIa and fXIa, despite their limited roles in hemostasis, are required for thrombosis in experimental animal models. If these proteins prove to be important contributors to thrombosis in humans, inhibiting them may produce an antithrombotic effect without significantly affecting hemostasis. The current understanding of the intrinsic pathway proteins in thrombosis in animal models and in human populations is discussed later.

THE INTRINSIC PATHWAY AND THROMBOSIS
Animal Models of Thrombosis

Mice lacking individual components of the intrinsic pathway, including the kallikrein-kinin system, have been tested for resistance to thrombus formation. FIX-deficient mice have a significant bleeding disorder (the murine equivalent of hemophilia B),[30] and are resistant to thrombus formation induced by injuring blood vessels with concentrated ferric chloride ($FeCl_3$).[30,31] In contrast, mice lacking fXI or fXII do not have obvious defects in hemostasis.[31–33] Despite this, counterintuitively, both fXI-deficient and fXII-deficient mice are as resistant to $FeCl_3$-induced thrombosis as are fIX-deficient mice.[31–33] The findings have been corroborated using a variety of other models and methods for inducing thrombosis,[33–35] and clearly indicate that an anticoagulant (antihemostatic) phenotype is not a prerequisite for an antithrombotic effect, at least under experimental conditions. More recent work has shown that

---

and natural compounds (often with a net negative charge), the plasma zymogens fXII and PK bind to the surface and reciprocally activate each other. Binding of PK is facilitated by the cofactor high-molecular-weight kininogen (HK). The process is probably triggered by traces of fXIIa or alpha-kallikrein present in plasma. Alpha-kallikrein can cleave HK to release the proinflammatory peptide bradykinin. The kallikrein-kinin may have several functions, including contributing to the innate immune response to microorganism invasion. Although fXIIa can initiate thrombin generation through the intrinsic pathway of coagulation (*yellow arrows*) by activating fXI, the kallikrein-kinin system does not seem to be required for hemostasis. Humans and other animals lacking fXII, PK, or HK do not have a bleeding disorder. However, there is mounting evidence that contact activation–induced coagulation through the intrinsic pathway may contribute to growth of pathologic clots during thrombosis. The nomenclature and symbols are the same as those used in (*A*). α-Kal; alpha-kallikrein.

mice lacking PK[35–37] or HK[38] are also resistant to injury-induced thrombus formation. Overall, these data imply that a process similar to classic contact activation may be driving thrombus formation through the intrinsic pathway in the mouse models.

Studies in primates have also shown roles for fXI and fXII in experimental thrombosis.[33,39–42] This work used inhibitory antibodies or antisense oligonucleotides (discussed later) to produce transient deficiency states. Thrombus formation was studied in prothrombotic collagen–coated or TF-coated vascular grafts inserted into temporary arteriovenous shunts in olive baboons (Papio anubis). In these studies the antithrombotic effect of fXI inhibition seemed to be greater than that of fXII inhibition.[33,40,41] A reduction in thrombus formation was detectable with as little as a 50% reduction in plasma fXI level,[42] with the maximum effect achieved at less than or equal to 20% of normal plasma concentration.

Although the data from the animal studies support the notion that the intrinsic pathway contributes to thrombosis, there are limitations to the preclinical analyses that must be considered. Because the animal species tested do not have natural propensities to form arterial or venous thrombi in the same manner as humans, vessels must be injured in some manner to produce a thrombus. Injury-induced thrombosis in an otherwise healthy, and usually young, animal may not mimic formation of thrombi in the diseased vessels of older humans.

Factor IX and Factor VIII in Thrombosis in Humans

FIX is the precursor of the protease fIXa, and activated fVIII (fVIIIa) is its cofactor. The severe bleeding disorders associated with deficiency of fIX (Hemophilia B) or fVIII (Hemophilia A) show their importance to hemostasis. There is a consistent correlation between plasma levels of fVIII in complex with von Willebrand factor (vWF) and risk for venous and arterial thrombosis in humans.[43–47] Supporting these observations, individuals with blood group O, who have 25% to 50% lower vWF and fVIII levels than individuals with a non-O blood group, are at lower risk for venous and arterial thrombosis.[48] High plasma levels of fIX are associated with modestly increased risks for venous thromboembolism (VTE), myocardial infarction (MI), and stroke.[49–53] These findings are supported by the impression that hemophiliacs have a lower risk of arterial thrombosis than nonhemophiliacs.[43,54]

Factor XI in Thrombosis in Humans

For fXI levels, the strongest correlations are with risk for VTE and ischemic stroke. The 10% of subjects in the Leiden Thrombophilia Study with the highest plasma fXI levels had a 2-fold higher risk of VTE compared with the lower 90%,[55] a result supported by recent data from the Longitudinal Investigation of Thromboembolism Etiology (LITE) cohort.[56] Consistent with these findings, fXI deficiency was associated with a reduced incidence of VTE in a study from Israel,[57] where severe deficiency is present in 1 in 450 individuals.[12,15] High plasma levels of fXI or fXIa were associated with increased risk for ischemic stroke in a study by Yang and colleagues,[58] in the Atherosclerosis Risk in Communities (ARIC) study,[53] and in the Risk of Arterial Thrombosis In relation to Oral contraceptives (RATIO) study.[59] Similarly, severe fXI deficiency was associated with a reduced incidence of stroke.[60]

A role for fXI in MI is not as clear as for VTE or stroke. Plasma fXI levels correlated with MI risk in men in the Study of Myocardial Infarction Leiden (SMILE),[51] and were higher in women with coronary disease than in women without it in a group undergoing cardiac catheterization.[61] However, fXI was not a risk factor for MI in the ARIC[53] or RATIO[59] studies, and fXIa levels were not linked to coronary disease in the second Northwick Park Heart Study (NPHS-II).[62] The incidence of MI in 96 individuals with severe fXI deficiency was similar to the expected incidence for age-matched controls.[63] The data are in line with recent work by Siegerink and colleagues[64] showing that an increased level of fXIa correlated more closely with risk for ischemic stroke than for MI in young women, and suggest that the contribution of fXI to thrombus formation is greater in some vascular beds than in others.

The Kallikrein-Kinin System in Thrombosis in Humans

Data supporting a role for fXII in VTE, stroke, or MI in humans are weak, and there is insufficient information to assess PK and HK. Note that congenital deficiency of C1-inhibitor (C1-INH), the major plasma regulator of fXIIa and alpha-kallikrein, causes hereditary angioedema, and does not seem to predispose to thrombosis.[26,27] FXII-deficient individuals are not protected from VTE,[65] and no differences in VTE incidences were noted across a range of fXII levels in LETS[66] and LITE[56] study participants. Data on fXII in arterial thrombosis are conflicting. FXII deficiency does not seem to protect individuals from stroke.[65] Plasma levels of fXIIa were inversely correlated with stroke risk in NPHS-II,[62] but were directly correlated with it in the RATIO study.[59] However, plasma fXII levels did not correlate with stroke risk in either study, or in the ARIC study.[53] In NPHS-II, increased fXIIa levels measured by specific enzyme-linked immunosorbent assay was associated with increased risk of MI, but fXIIa level measured as a complex with C1-INH indicated the opposite effect.[62] In the RATIO study, fXIIa, fXII, and PK levels were not associated with MI,[59] and risk of coronary events did not correlate with fXII in the ARIC study.[53] In addition, data from the SMILE cohort showed an inverse relationship between fXII levels and cardiovascular disease.[51] Endler and colleagues[67] also noted an inverse association between fXII and death from ischemic heart disease, although the relationship did not hold for severe fXII deficiency (<10% of normal), for which the risk was comparable with that of the population mean.

The Intrinsic Pathway and Thrombosis in Humans: Summary

Although it is difficult to draw firm conclusions from the complicated human epidemiologic data, it seems reasonable to conclude that the contribution of fXII to VTE, stroke, and MI in humans is probably smaller than for fXI and fIX. Although this conclusion conflicts with data from mouse models, in which fXII is a major contributor to thrombus formation, it is in reasonable agreement with results obtained in primates. It is possible that feedback activation of fXI by thrombin (see **Fig. 1**B) is stronger in primates than in mice, with fXIIa serving a smaller role in fXI activation. Another possibility is that a greater degree of fXIIa inhibition is required to produce an antithrombotic effect comparable with what is seen with fXIa inhibition in primates. These observations notwithstanding, there are situations in which fXIIa is likely to be a major driver of thrombosis in humans. For example, contact activation is triggered when blood is exposed to artificial surfaces during cardiopulmonary bypass[68,69] and extracorporeal membrane oxygenation (ECMO),[70] requiring full anticoagulation with heparin to prevent thrombotic complications.

TRIALS OF AGENTS TARGETING COMPONENTS OF THE INTRINSIC PATHWAY
Clinical Trials of Factor IXa Inhibitors

FIX seems to be an attractive target for antithrombotic therapy because of its role in sustaining thrombin generation, and its dual mode of activation through the extrinsic and intrinsic pathways. Patients with moderate or mild fIX deficiency (1%–5% and 6%–30% activity, respectively) generally experience bleeding only with trauma or surgery, suggesting that subtotal fIXa inhibition may be tolerated reasonably well.[14] This hypothesis is supported by preclinical studies showing potent antithrombotic effects for antibody, small molecule, and aptamer inhibitors of fIXa, with minimal bleeding.[71,72] However, the phenotype of complete fIX deficiency (severe Hemophilia B), which includes spontaneous bleeding into joints and soft tissues,[14] indicates that there are limits to the intensity of therapeutic inhibition of fIXa. Human studies of fIXa inhibitors have been limited to testing the small molecule TTP889, and the RNA aptamer systems REG1and REG2.[73]

TTP889 is an orally available small molecule that partially inhibits fIXa activity (maximum ~90%).[73] In animal studies the drug had efficacy against venous and arterial thrombosis.[74] At what were considered supratherapeutic concentrations, TTP889 did not affect the aPTT. This finding contrasts with other types of fIXa inhibitor, which prolong the aPTT in animal models. TTP889 was tested in a randomized placebo-controlled study as extended prophylaxis for VTE in patients who had undergone hip fracture repair followed by standard prophylaxis for 5 to 9 days.[72] Rates of VTE, as determined by venography, were similar in the TTP889 and placebo groups after 3 weeks of therapy. This finding, and the fact that there were no differences in major bleeding, raised concerns that TTP889 was inadequately dosed. A phase II trial of TTP889 in patients undergoing ventricular assist device implantation was terminated early, and the drug has not been assessed further.

RNA aptamers are single-stranded oligonucleotides that bind to a target of interest.[75] They are selected for specific functional capabilities from pools of random RNA sequences. Aptamers can be regulated with a complementary oligonucleotide that neutralizes activity through Watson-Crick base pairing. The REG1 and REG2 systems are composed of parenterally administered aptamers that target fIXa.[73] REG1 includes the inhibitory aptamer RB006 (pegnivacogin) and its complement RB007 (anivamersen), both formulated for intravenous administration. REG2 is a formulation of RB006 for subcutaneous administration, with RB007 as its reversal agent. In phase 1 studies involving single and repeat escalating doses in healthy volunteers, RB006 showed quick onset of action with significant fIXa inhibition.[76,77] Although phase 2 studies showed the feasibility of using the REG1 system in patients with coronary artery disease,[78,79] the RADAR phase 2b trial in patients with acute coronary syndrome was stopped early because of serious allergic reactions.[79] In a phase III trial of patients with acute coronary syndrome undergoing percutaneous coronary intervention, REG1 seemed to be comparable with bivalirudin in reducing the incidence of ischemic events.[80] However the statistical power of the study was limited because it was stopped early, again because of allergic side effects. Therapy-related bleeding was also a concern: 0.4% of patients receiving REG1 had severe or fatal bleeding compared with 0.1% of patients receiving bivalirudin, and the rate of moderate to severe bleeding was also significantly higher in the REG1 group.[80]

The experience with fIXa inhibitors shows the challenge of producing an adequate antithrombotic effect by targeting a protease that serves a major role in hemostasis. The therapeutic window may be narrow. The partial inhibition of fIXa achievable with TTP889 was inadequate to prevent thrombus formation in patients with coronary disease, whereas the greater inhibition achieved with REG1 led to an increase in bleeding events compared with standard therapy. The limited data are not sufficient to fully assess the utility of inhibiting fIXa as an antithrombotic strategy in humans. However, the data that are available raise the possibility that it may be more difficult to achieve a reproducible, effective, and safe antithrombotic effect with a fIXa inhibitor than with inhibitors of fXa or thrombin.

Antisense-induced Reduction of Factor XI Levels

Modified DNA antisense oligonucleotides (ASOs), or gapmers, have been widely used in research to specifically reduce expression of a protein of interest in vivo.[81] In contrast with the RNA aptamers described earlier, which directly inhibit coagulation in plasma, ASOs interfere with intracellular synthesis of a target protein. After entering a cell, the ASO binds through complementary base pairing to a specific mRNA, leading to its selective degradation and reduced synthesis of the encoded protein. Second-generation gapmers are avidly taken up by hepatocytes, facilitating targeting of coagulation factors. Their long tissue elimination half-lives allow administration at intervals of several days to weeks.

The ASO ISIS-416858 (now IONIS-416858) is complementary to a sequence in the human and rhesus macaque fXI mRNA.[82] In a phase I study, volunteers received 3 subcutaneous doses (50–300 mg) of ISIS-416858 during the first week of therapy, followed by weekly doses.[83] Those receiving 200-mg and 300-mg doses had, on average, ~80% reduction in plasma fXI level, with greater than 95% reduction achieved in some individuals. Plasma fXI levels remained well below baseline for several weeks after the last dose. There was no excessive bleeding, nor was there evidence of significant liver, kidney, or blood cell abnormalities in study subjects. Mild irritation at injection sites was the most common side effect.

In a phase 2 randomized trial, ISIS-416858 was compared with standard-dose low-molecular-weight heparin as prophylaxis to prevent VTE in patients undergoing knee replacement.[84] The ASO was given in 200-mg or 300-mg doses on study days 1, 3, 5, 8, 15, 22, and 29, with surgery on day 36. Additional doses were given on the day of surgery, and 3 days postsurgery (day 39). Patients randomized to enoxaparin received the first dose the evening before surgery or 6 to 8 hours after surgery, and then once daily for at least 8 days. On the day of surgery, average plasma fXI levels were 38% and 20% of normal in patients on the 200-mg or 300-mg ASO doses, respectively, and 93% in patients on enoxaparin. Several patients receiving the ASO had fXI levels less than 5% of normal. Bilateral lower extremity venography performed 8 to 12 days postsurgery detected thrombi in 30% of enoxaparin-treated patients, 27% of patients on the 200-mg ASO dose, and 4% on the 300-mg ASO dose. The incidence of VTE was 5% in individuals from the 2 ASO groups with plasma fXI levels of less than or equal to 20% of normal at the time of surgery. There were few symptomatic clots in any treatment group (2 in the 200 mg ASO group and 1 in the enoxaparin group). Although there was no placebo group in this study, venographically detectable thrombi would be expected in ~45% of untreated patients undergoing knee replacement.[85] Clinically relevant bleeding occurred in 3% of patients on ASOs and 8% on enoxaparin.

There are several notable results from this study. First, 300-mg ISIS-416858 was superior to enoxaparin for reducing VTE. Although the fVIIa/TF complex is thought to play a major role in VTE during orthopedic surgery,[86] this result raises the possibility that a fXI-dependent pathway dominates the process during knee replacement. Thrombi that formed in the 300-mg ASO group were not only rarer but considerably smaller than thrombi in patients receiving 200-mg ASO or enoxaparin.[84] This response mirrors results from primate studies with ISIS-416858 showing that reduction of fXI level to 20% of normal is associated with a better antithrombotic effect than a reduction to 50% of normal.[42] In addition, because of the mechanism of action, ASO treatment was started 5 weeks before surgery, and patients were under the full drug effect during surgery. Despite this, abnormal hemostasis was not observed intraoperatively, even in patients with fXI levels less than 5% of normal, and postoperative bleeding was rare. This finding shows the safety of reducing fXI levels in this setting, and supports the hypothesis that it is possible to dissociate an antithrombotic effect from a major effect on hemostasis, at least in some situations.

Targeting the Kallikrein-Kinin System

Although protein (ecallantide) and small molecule (BCX7353 and BCX4161) plasma kallikrein inhibitors have been used to treat idiopathic and hereditary angioedema, inhibition of fXIIa or alpha-kallikrein has not been tested in humans for treatment or prevention of thrombosis. Epidemiologic data do not support a role for fXII in common conditions such as VTE, stroke, and MI; however, there are situations in which contact activation likely contributes to thrombosis. As discussed, contact activation occurs during cardiopulmonary bypass[68,69] and ECMO,[70] during which blood is exposed to artificial surfaces for prolonged periods. In a rabbit-ECMO model, the anti-fXIIa monoclonal immunoglobulin G 3F7 was as effective as heparin in preventing thrombus formation in the extracorporeal circuit.[87,88] As expected, 3F7 did not compromise hemostasis, whereas heparin produced a significant bleeding propensity. Another potential advantage of a fXIIa inhibitor in this setting is that it would inhibit PK activation, blunting bradykinin production and reducing inflammation (see **Fig. 1**C). In rabbits in which thrombus formation is induced by intravenous placement of polyurethane catheters, ASO-induced depletion of fXII or fXI was more effective at maintaining vessel patency than fVII depletion.[89] Thus, inhibitors of fXIIa may be useful replacements or adjuncts for drugs such as heparin and warfarin in clinic scenarios in which blood is exposed to nonbiological materials. A variety of compounds targeting fXIIa (reviewed in Ref.[90]) are undergoing preclinical testing, and should be available for clinical testing in the near future.

SUMMARY

The cascade-waterfall hypothesis of intrinsic blood coagulation has served as the foundation for tests used in clinical practice for more than 50 years.[10,11] Although models based on this hypothesis, such as a the one shown in **Fig. 1**A, accurately described the manner in which plasma clots in in vitro assays such as the aPTT, the clinical presentations of patients lacking various plasma factors involved in the cascade make it clear that the traditional intrinsic pathway is not an accurate representation of the processes that stop bleeding at a wound site. This realization has led to revisions, such as those shown in **Fig. 1**B, that are in better agreement with clinical observations.[12,17] The bleeding tendencies seen in genetically altered mice lacking components of the plasma coagulation mechanism, in general, support the revised model for hemostasis.[20] However, work over the past decade with animal models also points to the possibility that a process more similar to the classic intrinsic pathway contributes to pathologic thrombin generation and raises the prospect that thrombosis might be treatable by targeting plasma factors that serve minor roles in hemostasis. If therapies directed at proteases, such as fXIa or fXIIa, are effective at treating or preventing thrombosis, the safety profile of antithrombotic therapy could be substantially improved. The recent demonstration that ASO-mediated reduction of fXI level is effective and safe for prevention of VTE in patients undergoing knee replacement surgery provides proof of concept for this premise.[84]

It is not certain why thrombus formation depends on fXI and fXII in some situations, but available data offer some clues. In the mouse and primate studies discussed earlier, inhibition of fXI or fXII did not prevent initial formation of clot on an injured vessel or thrombogenic surface, but had a dramatic effect on propagation of clot growth away from the vessel wall into the lumen.[31–34,39–41] Intraluminal thrombi forming in the absence of fXI or fXII are unstable, and fragment under the shear stresses in flowing blood. During hemostasis after vessel injury, clot forms primarily outside the damaged blood vessel and within the blood vessel wall. Thrombus growth into the vessel lumen is probably not required to achieve hemostasis. The shear forces produced by flowing blood would be high within the blood vessel lumen, and would increase as the lumen narrows from a growing intraluminal thrombus. Under these circumstances, the intrinsic pathway may support thrombin generation on the surface of the thrombus that maintains its stability and promotes its growth. We need to identify the factors that promote activation of intrinsic pathway proteases during thrombosis to better understand these processes.

A variety of compounds targeting fXI and fXIa have undergone preclinical testing and some have entered phase 1 studies.[90] Going forward, it seems reasonable to initially test fXI/fXIa inhibitors for prevention of thrombosis. At this point, there is insufficient information to predict whether inhibition of intrinsic pathway components would be suitable for treatment of acute thrombotic processes. Based on the epidemiologic data, prevention of VTE and stroke should both be considered.[55–60] The results of the ASO knee replacement trial raise the possibility that fXIa inhibition is superior to current standard of care for preventing postoperative DVT.[84] Larger trials are needed to conclusively show this, and to adequately assess differences in bleeding risk. The phase 2 ASO knee replacement trial was not powered sufficiently to evaluate bleeding.[84] Inhibition of fXI may be a particularly attractive option for secondary VTE prevention. The strategy of extending anticoagulation therapy beyond the typical 3 to 6 months for treatment of an unprovoked deep vein thrombus or pulmonary embolus is being actively debated.[91,92] Prevention of rare fatal events by extending prophylaxis may be offset by the increased risk of major bleeding episodes. However, prevention of common complications of VTE that have a major impact on quality of life, such as postthrombotic syndrome and pulmonary hypertension, may warrant extended treatment. The fXI ASO trials suggest that targeted fXI inhibition would be associated with a lower bleeding risk than with warfarin, or an oral thrombin or fXa inhibitor. Inhibiting fXIa may also be useful for primary or secondary prevention in patients with atrial fibrillation or other high-risk conditions who are not good candidates for conventional anticoagulation because of comorbidities, or as short-term prophylaxis after neurosurgery or other procedures in which even modest anticoagulant-induced bleeding must be avoided.

Given the likely favorable safety profiles of inhibitors of fXIa and fXIIa, it may be possible to add such compounds to current standards of care to enhance therapeutic benefit without appreciably changing bleeding risk. FXI-deficient patients have been treated safely with warfarin or antiplatelet therapy, suggesting that this approach would be safe.[93] It is also possible that fXIa or fXIIa inhibitors may allow doses of other antithrombotic drugs to be reduced, reducing the overall bleeding risk. FXIa and fXIIa inhibitors may have an advantage compared with current anticoagulants in situations in which contact activation is triggered by exposure of blood to artificial surfaces such as extracorporeal circuits and indwelling intravascular devices.[68–70,87–89] The recent work showing that fXIIa inhibition prevents thrombus formation in experimental ECMO[87,88] suggests that inhibitors of fXIIa or fXIa may be able to replace or supplement heparin in patients on extracorporeal circuits. There is also a need for alternatives to warfarin for patients with mechanical heart valves. Although the contributions of fXIa and fXIIa to thrombus formation induced by mechanical heart valves have not been evaluated, there is evidence that components of such valves can induce contact activation in plasma.[94]

With the demonstration that therapeutic manipulation of fXI can produce a potent antithrombotic effect in humans, future work should focus on establishing the clinical scenarios in which fXI and fXII contribute to thrombosis, and determining the optimal target for each situation. If drugs directed at these proteases show efficacy in clinical trials, their safety profiles should widen the spectrum of conditions in which antithrombotic therapy can be administered, and increase the number of patients who are eligible for antithrombotic therapy.

REFERENCES

1. Crawley JT, Zanardelli S, Chion CK, et al. The central role of thrombin in hemostasis. J Thromb Haemost 2007;5(Suppl 1):95–101.
2. Yeh CH, Hogg K, Weitz JI. Overview of the new oral anticoagulants: opportunities and challenges. Arterioscler Thromb Vasc Biol 2015;35:1056–65.
3. Mulloy B, Hogwood J, Gray E, et al. Pharmacology of heparin and related drugs. Pharmacol Rev 2016;68:76–141.
4. Ageno W, Gallus AS, Wittkosky A, et al. Oral anticoagulation therapy: antithrombotic therapy and prevention of thrombosis, 9th ed: American College of Chest Physicians evidence-based clinical practice guidelines. Chest 2012;141(Suppl 2):e44S–88S.
5. Crowther MA, Warkentin TE. Bleeding risk and the management of bleeding complications in patients undergoing anticoagulant therapy: focus on new anticoagulant agents. Blood 2008;111:4871–9.
6. Chai-Adisaksopha C, Crowther M, Isayama T, et al. The impact of bleeding complications in patients receiving target-specific oral anticoagulants: a systematic review and meta-analysis. Blood 2014;124:2450–8.
7. Kenne E, Nickel KF, Long AT, et al. Factor XII: a novel target for safe prevention of thrombosis and inflammation. J Intern Med 2015;278:571–85.
8. Chen Z, Seiffert D, Hawes B. Inhibition of factor XI activity as a promising antithrombotic strategy. Drug Discov Today 2014;19:1435–9.
9. Gailani D, Bane CE, Gruber A. Factor XI and contact activation as targets for antithrombotic therapy. J Thromb Haemost 2015;13:1383–95.
10. Macfarlane RG. An enzyme cascade in the blood clotting mechanism, and its function as a biochemical amplifier. Nature 1964;202:498–9.
11. Davie EW, Ratnoff OD. Waterfall sequence for intrinsic blood coagulation. Science 1964;145:1310–2.
12. Gailani D, Neff AT. Rare coagulation factor deficiencies. In: Hoffman R, Benz EJ, Silberstein LE, et al, editors. Hematology: basic principles and practice. 6th edition. Philadelphia: Saunders-Elsevier; 2013. p. 1971–86.
13. Wolberg AS, Mast AE. Tissue factor and factor VIIa – hemostasis and beyond. Thromb Res 2012;129(Suppl 2):S1–4.
14. Carcao M, Moorehead P, Lillicrap D. Hemophilia A and B. In: Hoffman R, Benz EJ, Silberstein LE, et al, editors. Hematology: basic principles and practice. 6th edition. Philadelphia: Saunders-Elsevier; 2013. p. 1940–60.
15. Duga S, Salomon O. Congenital factor XI deficiency: an update. Semin Thromb Hemost 2013;39:621–31.
16. James P, Salomon O, Mikovic D, et al. Rare bleeding disorders – bleeding assessment tools, laboratory aspects and phenotype and therapy of FXI deficiency. Haemophilia 2014;20(Suppl 4):71–5.
17. Broze GJ. Tissue factor pathway inhibitor and the revised theory of coagulation. Annu Rev Med 1995;46:103–12.

18. Mackman N. The role of tissue factor and factor VIIa in hemostasis. Anesth Analg 2009;108:1447–52.
19. Doolittle RF. Step-by-step evolution of vertebrate coagulation. Cold Spring Harb Symp Quant Biol 2009;74:35–40.
20. McManus MP, Gailani D. Mouse models of coagulation factor deficiencies, in animal models of diseases: translational medicine perspective for drug discovery and development. Bentham Scientific Publishers; 2012. p. 67–121.
21. Ponczek MB, Gailani D, Doolittle RF. Evolution of the contact phase of vertebrate blood coagulation. J Thromb Haemost 2008;6:1876–83.
22. Emsley J, McEwan PA, Gailani D. Structure and function of factor XI. Blood 2010; 115:2569–77.
23. Naito K, Fujikawa K. Activation of human blood coagulation factor XI independent of factor XII. Factor XI is activated by thrombin and factor XIa in the presence of negatively charged surfaces. J Biol Chem 1991;266:7353–8.
24. Gailani D, Broze GJ Jr. Factor XI activation in a revised model of blood coagulation. Science 1991;253:909–12.
25. Matafonov A, Sarilla S, Sun MF, et al. Activation of factor XI by products of prothrombin activation. Blood 2011;118:437–45.
26. Long AT, Kenne E, Jung R, et al. Contact system revisited: an interface between inflammation, coagulation, and innate immunity. J Thromb Haemost 2016;14(3): 427–37.
27. Schmaier AH. The contact activation and kallikrein/kinin systems: pathophysiologic and physiologic activities. J Thromb Haemost 2016;14:28–39.
28. Frick IM, Björck L, Herwald H. The dual role of the contact system in bacterial infectious disease. Thromb Haemost 2007;98:497–502.
29. Frick IM, Akesson P, Herwald H, et al. The contact system – a novel branch of innate immunity generating antibacterial peptides. EMBO J 2006;25:5569–78.
30. Lin HF, Maeda N, Smithies O, et al. A coagulation factor IX-deficient mouse model for human hemophilia B. Blood 1997;90:3962–6.
31. Wang X, Cheng Q, Xu L, et al. Effects of factor IX or factor XI deficiency on ferric chloride-induced carotid artery occlusion in mice. J Thromb Haemost 2005;3: 695–702.
32. Renné T, Pozgajová M, Grüner S, et al. Defective thrombus formation in mice lacking coagulation factor XII. J Exp Med 2005;202:271–81.
33. Cheng Q, Tucker EI, Pine MS, et al. A role for factor XIIa-mediated factor XI activation in thrombus formation in vivo. Blood 2010;116:3981–9.
34. Müller F, Mutch NJ, Schenk WA, et al. Platelet polyphosphates are proinflammatory and procoagulant mediators in vivo. Cell 2009;139:1143–56.
35. Revenko AS, Gao D, Crosby JR, et al. Selective depletion of plasma prekallikrein or coagulation factor XII inhibits thrombosis in mice without increased bleeding. Blood 2011;188:5302–11.
36. Bird JE, Smith PL, Wang X, et al. Effects of plasma kallikrein deficiency on haemostasis and thrombosis in mice: murine ortholog of the Fletcher trait. Thromb Haemost 2012;107:1141–50.
37. Stavrou EX, Fang C, Merkulova A, et al. Reduced thrombosis in Klkb1-/- mice is mediated by increased Mas receptor, prostacyclin, Sirt1, and KLF4 and decreased tissue factor. Blood 2015;125:710–9.
38. Merkulov S, Zhang WM, Komar AA, et al. Deletion of murine kininogen gene 1 (mKng1) causes loss of plasma kininogen and delays thrombosis. Blood 2008; 111:1274–81.

39. Gruber A, Hanson SR. Factor XI-dependence of surface- and tissue factor-initiated thrombus propagation in primates. Blood 2003;102:953–5.
40. Tucker EI, Marzec UM, White TC, et al. Prevention of vascular graft occlusion and thrombus-associated thrombin generation by inhibition of factor XI. Blood 2009; 113:936–44.
41. Matafonov A, Leung PY, Gailani AE, et al. Factor XII inhibition reduces thrombus formation in a primate thrombosis model. Blood 2014;123:1739–46.
42. Crosby JR, Marzec U, Revenko AS, et al. Antithrombotic effect of antisense factor XI oligonucleotide treatment in primates. Arterioscler Thromb Vasc Biol 2013;33: 1670–8.
43. Lowe G. Factor IX and deep vein thrombosis. Haematologica 2009;94:615–7.
44. Bertina RM. Elevated clotting factor levels and venous thrombosis. Pathophysiol Haemost Thromb 2003;33:395–400.
45. Rumley A, Lowe GD, Sweetnam PM, et al. Factor VIII, von Willebrand factor and the risk of major ischaemic heart disease in the Caerphilly Study. Br J Haematol 1999;105:110–6.
46. Whincup P, Danesh J, Walker M, et al. Von Willebrand factor and coronary heart disease: prospective study and meta-analysis. Eur Heart J 2002;23:1764–70.
47. Tsai AW, Cushman M, Rosamond WD, et al. Coagulation factors, inflammation markers, and venous thromboembolism: the Longitudinal Investigation of Thromboembolism Etiology (LITE). Am J Med 2002;113:636–42.
48. Wu O, Bayoumi N, Vickers MA, et al. ABO (H) blood groups and vascular disease: a systematic review and meta-analysis. J Thromb Haemost 2008;6:62–9.
49. van Hylckama Vlieg A, van der Linden IK, Bertina RM, et al. High levels of factor IX increase the risk of venous thrombosis. Blood 2000;95:3678–82.
50. Heikal NM, Murphy KK, Crist RA, et al. Elevated factor IX activity is associated with an increased odds ratio for both arterial and venous thrombotic events. Am J Clin Pathol 2013;140:680–5.
51. Doggen CJ, Rosendaal FR, Meijers JC. Levels of intrinsic coagulation factors and the risk of myocardial infarction among men: opposite and synergistic effects of factors XI and XII. Blood 2006;108:4045–51.
52. Tanis B, Algra A, van der Graaf Y, et al. Procoagulant factors and the risk of myocardial infarction in young women. Eur Heart J 2006;77:67–73.
53. Suri MF, Yamagishi K, Aleksic N, et al. Novel hemostatic factor levels and risk of ischemic stroke: the Atherosclerosis Risk in Communities (ARIC) Study. Cerebrovasc Dis 2010;29:497–502.
54. Sramek A, Kriek M, Rosendaal FR. Decreased mortality of ischaemic heart disease among carriers of haemophilia. Lancet 2003;362:351–4.
55. Meijers JC, Tekelenburg WL, Bouma BN, et al. High levels of coagulation factor XI as a risk factor for venous thrombosis. N Engl J Med 2000;342:696–701.
56. Cushman M, O'Meara ES, Folsom AR, et al. Coagulation factors IX through XIII and the risk of future venous thrombosis: the longitudinal investigation of thromboembolism etiology. Blood 2009;114:2878–83.
57. Salomon O, Steinberg DM, Zucker M, et al. Patients with severe factor XI deficiency have a reduced incidence of deep-vein thrombosis. Thromb Haemost 2011;105:269–73.
58. Yang DT, Flanders MM, Kim H, et al. Elevated factor XI activity levels are associated with an increased odds ratio for cerebrovascular events. Am J Clin Pathol 2006;126:411–5.
59. Siegerink B, Govers-Riemslag JW, Rosendaal FR, et al. Intrinsic coagulation activation and the risk of arterial thrombosis in young women: results from the Risk of

Arterial Thrombosis in Relation to Oral Contraceptives (RATIO) case-control study. Circulation 2010;122:1854–61.

60. Salomon O, Steinberg DM, Koren-Morag N, et al. Reduced incidence of ischemic stroke in patients with severe factor XI deficiency. Blood 2008;111:4113–7.

61. Berliner JI, Rybicki AC, Kaplan RC, et al. Elevated levels of factor XI are associated with cardiovascular disease in women. Thromb Res 2002;107:55–60.

62. Govers-Riemslag JW, Smid M, Cooper JA, et al. The plasma kallikrein-kinin system and risk of cardiovascular disease in men. J Thromb Haemost 2007;5:1896–903.

63. Salomon O, Steinberg DM, Dardik R, et al. Inherited factor XI deficiency confers no protection against acute myocardial infarction. J Thromb Haemost 2003;1:658–61.

64. Siegerink B, Maino A, Algra A, et al. Hypercoagulability and the risk of myocardial infarction and ischemic stroke in young woman. J Thromb Haemost 2015;13:1568–75.

65. Zeerleder S, Schloesser M, Redondo M. Reevaluation of the incidence of thromboembolic complications in congenital factor XII deficiency–a study on 73 subjects from 14 Swiss families. Thromb Haemost 1999;82:1240–6.

66. Koster T, Rosendaal FR, Briet E, et al. John Hageman's factor and deep-vein thrombosis: Leiden Thrombophilia Study. Br J Haematol 1994;87:422–4.

67. Endler G, Marsik C, Jilma B, et al. Evidence of a U-shaped association between factor XII activity and overall survival. J Thromb Haemost 2007;5:1143–8.

68. Sonntag J, Dähnert I, Stiller B, et al. Complement and contact activation during cardiovascular operations in infants. Ann Thorac Surg 1998;65:525–31.

69. Wendel HP, Jones DW, Gallimore MJ. FXII levels, FXIIa-like activities and kallikrein activities in normal subjects and patients undergoing cardiac surgery. Immunopharmacology 1999;45:141–4.

70. Plötz FB, van Oeveren W, Bartlett RH, et al. Blood activation during neonatal extracorporeal life support. J Thorac Cardiovasc Surg 1993;105:823–32.

71. Howard EL, Becker KC, Rusconi CP, et al. Factor IXa inhibitors as novel anticoagulants. Arterioscler Thromb Vasc Biol 2007;27:722–7.

72. Eriksson BI, Dahl OE, Lassen MR, et al. Partial factor IXa inhibition with TTP889 for prevention of venous thromboembolism: an exploratory study. J Thromb Haemost 2008;6:457–63.

73. Eikelboom JW, Zelenkofske SL, Rusconi CP. Coagulation factor IXa as a target for treatment and prophylaxis of venous thromboembolism. Arterioscler Thromb Vasc Biol 2010;30:382–7.

74. Rothlein R, Shen JM, Naser N, et al. TTP889, a novel orally active partial inhibitor of FIXa inhibits clotting in two a/v shunt models without prolonging bleeding times. Blood 2005;106:A1886.

75. Woodruff RS, Sullenger BA. Modulation of the coagulation cascade using aptamers. Arterioscler Thromb Vasc Biol 2015;35:2083–91.

76. Dyke CK, Steinhubl SR, Kleiman NS, et al. First-in-human experience of an antidote-controlled anticoagulant using RNA aptamer technology: a phase 1a pharmacodynamic evaluation of a drug-antidote pair for the controlled regulation of factor IXa activity. Circulation 2006;114:2490–7.

77. Chan MY, Rusconi CP, Alexander JH, et al. A randomized, repeat-dose, pharmacodynamic and safety study of an antidote-controlled factor IXa inhibitor. J Thromb Haemost 2008;6:789–96.

78. Cohen MG, Purdy DA, Rossi JS, et al. First clinical application of an actively reversible direct factor IXa inhibitor as an anticoagulation strategy in patients undergoing percutaneous coronary intervention. Circulation 2010;122:614–22.
79. Povsic TJ, Vavalle JP, Aberle LH, et al. A Phase 2, randomized, partially blinded, active-controlled study assessing the efficacy and safety of variable anticoagulation reversal using the REG1 system in patients with acute coronary syndromes: results of the RADAR trial. Eur Heart J 2013;34:2481–9.
80. Lincoff AM, Mehran R, Povsic TJ, et al. Effect of the REG1 anticoagulation system versus bivalirudin on outcomes after percutaneous coronary intervention (REGULATE-PCI): a randomized clinical trial. Lancet 2016;387(10016):349–56.
81. Zhang H, Löwenberg EC, Crosby JR, et al. Inhibition of the intrinsic coagulation pathway factor XI by antisense oligonucleotides: a novel antithrombotic strategy with lowered bleeding risk. Blood 2010;116:4684–92.
82. Younis HS, Crosby J, Huh JI, et al. Antisense inhibition of coagulation factor XI prolongs APTT without increased bleeding risk in cynomolgus monkeys. Blood 2012;119:2401–8.
83. Liu Q, Bethune C, Dessouki E, et al. ISIS-FXI$_{Rx}$, a novel and specific antisense inhibitor of factor XI, caused significant reduction in FXI antigen and activity and increased aPTT without causing bleeding in healthy volunteers. Blood 2011;118:A209.
84. Büller HR, Bethune C, Bhanot S, et al. Factor XI antisense oligonucleotide for prevention of venous thrombosis. N Engl J Med 2015;372:232–40.
85. Fuji T, Fujita S, Tachibana S, et al. A dose-ranging study evaluating the oral factor Xa inhibitor edoxaban for the prevention of venous thromboembolism in patients undergoing total knee arthroplasty. J Thromb Haemost 2010;8:2458–68.
86. Owens AP 3rd, Mackman N. Tissue factor and thrombosis: the clot starts here. Thromb Haemost 2010;104:432–9.
87. Larsson M, Rayzman V, Nolte MW, et al. A factor XIIa inhibitory antibody provides thromboprotection in extracorporeal circulation without increasing bleeding risk. Sci Transl Med 2014;6:222ra17.
88. Worm M, Köhler EC, Panda R, et al. The factor XIIa blocking antibody 3F7: a safe anticoagulant with anti-inflammatory activities. Ann Transl Med 2015;3:247.
89. Yau JW, Liao P, Fredenburgh JC, et al. Selective depletion of factor XI or factor XII with antisense oligonucleotides attenuates catheter thrombosis in rabbits. Blood 2014;123:2102–7.
90. Gailani D. Future prospects for contact factors as therapeutic targets. Hematology Am Soc Hematol Educ Program 2014;2014:52–9.
91. Schulman S. Secondary prevention of venous thromboembolism. BMJ 2013;347: f5440.
92. Kearson C, Akl EA. Duration of anticoagulant therapy for deep vein thrombosis and pulmonary embolism. Blood 2013;123:1794–801.
93. Salomon O, Seligsohn U. New observations on factor XI deficiency. Haemophilia 2004;10(Suppl 4):184–7.
94. Jaffer IH, Fredenburgh JC, Hirsh J, et al. Medical device-induced thrombosis: what causes it and how can we prevent it? J Thromb Haemost 2015;13(Suppl 1):S72–81.

Regulatory Impact on Thrombosis Treatment, Prevention, and Anticoagulant Use

Robert Dannemiller, PharmD, Tucker Ward,
John Fanikos, RPh, MBA*

KEYWORDS

- Venous thromboembolism • Stroke • Anticoagulation • Regulatory affairs
- Health policy

KEY POINTS

- Anticoagulants are a high-risk class of medications and are subject to oversight by many regulatory agencies through collaborative efforts.
- Use of electronic health records can improve patient care by providing clinicians with updated health information.
- Nationwide efforts are being developed and implemented to improve quality of care and limit the number of adverse drug events associated with anticoagulant drug therapy.

INTRODUCTION

Anticoagulation is the cornerstone therapy for thrombosis treatment and prevention. Atrial fibrillation (AF) increases the risk of thromboembolic stroke five-fold. The number of patients afflicted is projected to reach 12 million in the United States by 2050 with health care expenditures estimated to increase to $2.2 trillion.[1,2] The diagnostic frequency of new and recurrent venous thromboembolism (VTE) is increasing. Corresponding resource use is expected to reach $69.3 billion in annual costs to the health care system.[3,4] Anticoagulant use is expected to grow for these and other conditions. Anticoagulants are considered high-risk medications. Adverse events with their use are common, often further complicate patient care, lead to higher costs, and compromise trust in providers.[5,6] Within the US government the Department of

Funding Source: None.
Disclosures: All authors have no disclosures related to this article.
Department of Pharmacy Services, Brigham and Women's Hospital, 75 Francis Street, Boston, MA 02115, USA
* Corresponding author.
E-mail address: JFanikos@partners.org

Hematol Oncol Clin N Am 30 (2016) 1115–1135
http://dx.doi.org/10.1016/j.hoc.2016.06.003
0889-8588/16/$ – see front matter © 2016 Elsevier Inc. All rights reserved.

hemonc.theclinics.com

Health and Human Services (HHS) is responsible for the delivery of health care and therefore has a stake in fostering advances in medicine, public health, and social services (**Fig. 1**). Several government agencies exist to regulate and support health care systems. Several nonprofit national organizations exist to communicate and serve as a catalyst for practice change. They have targeted thromboembolism and anticoagulants to improve patient outcomes and enhance safety because many communications have either a delayed or limited impact on clinician behavior and use of health system resources.[7–9]

This article reviews regulatory and agency efforts related to thromboembolic disease and anticoagulant management with the intent of updating clinicians and highlighting the implications for practice.

OVERVIEW OF ORGANIZATION INTERACTIONS AND PERFORMANCE MEASURES

Nonprofit national organizations, professional organizations, and government agencies work collaboratively to establish evidence-based consensus standards for best practice and develop performance measures to ensure quality health care delivery (**Table 1**). In 1998, the Joint Commission's (TJC) introduced the first national quality measurement program and reporting became mandatory for accreditation in 2002.[10] In the time period since, the National Quality Forum and the Centers for Medicare and Medicaid Services (CMS) endorsed and introduced additional quality measures as part of the Hospital Inpatient Quality Reporting (IQR) Program. Beginning in 2004, CMS began withholding payments for hospitals that did not report TJC quality measures to CMS. Many of these are directed at anticoagulation use for thrombosis prevention and treatment (**Table 2**).

TJC has implemented several changes to the performance measure requirements.[11] These efforts were designed to provide hospitals with greater flexibility and to further align TJC reporting standards with those of CMS. Today most health care institutions collect performance measures through a quality department, often with assistance from a survey or analytics vendor.[12] There is a choice of measures to report, with the stipulation that these measures are applicable to the services provided and patient populations served by the hospital. Institutions may report using

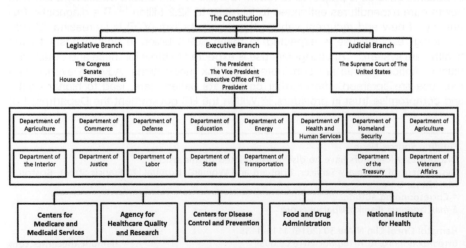

Fig. 1. US government agencies supporting health care systems.

Table 1
Government and nonprofit agencies impacting health care

Organization	Description	Goals and Focus	Measurements
The National Quality Forum	Nonprofit, nonpartisan, membership-based organization that works to catalyze improvements in healthcare.	Convenes working groups to foster quality improvement in public and private sectors.	Endorses consensus standards for performance measurement.
The Joint Commission	Nonprofit organization that accredits health care organizations and certifies programs in the United States.	Sets standards and objectively evaluates processes to measure, assess, and improve performance at the following: Hospitals: general, children's, psychiatric, rehabilitation Home care: medical equipment services, pharmacy, hospice services Nursing care: nursing homes, rehabilitation centers Ambulatory care: group practices, office-based surgery practices Laboratory: independent or freestanding clinical laboratories	The standards focus on critical patient care and organization functions that are essential to providing safe, high-quality care. Each standard is reasonable, achievable, and measurable and expectations for organization performance.
Centers for Medicare and Medicaid Services	Federal agency within the US Department of Health and Human Services that administers the Medicare program and works in partnership with state governments to administer Medicaid program.	The Medicare Prescription Drug, Improvement, and Modernization Act of 2003 mandated the Hospital Inpatient Quality Reporting program. This authorized Centers for Medicare and Medicaid Services to pay hospitals that successfully report designated quality measures at higher payment rates, giving hospitals a financial incentive to report the quality of their services.	Hospital quality of care information gathered through the program is available to consumers on the Hospital Compare Web site at: www. hospitalcompare.hhs.gov.
Agency for Health Quality and Research	Federal agency within the Department of Health and Human Services that supports research on improving health care quality.	Uses a system of quality indicators to determine the standards of quality health care and if a particular provider is meeting those standards.	Indicators that monitor different aspects of health care quality: • Prevention Quality Indicator: identifies hospital readmissions that could have been avoided. • In-patient Quality Indicator: identifies patient mortality rates in-hospital caused by lack of care or surgical procedures. • Patient Safety Indicators: identifies avoidable complications.

Table 2
National hospital inpatient quality indicators and performance measures: examples impacting thrombosis treatment and prevention

TJC Identifier	NQF Identifier	Description	Measurement
SCIP VTE 2	NQF 0218	Surgery patients who received appropriate VTE prophylaxis within 24 hours prior to surgery to 24 hours after surgery.	Surgery patients who received appropriate VTE prophylaxis within 24 hours prior to anesthesia start time to 24 hours after anesthesia end time divided by all selected surgery patients.
VTE 1	NQF 0371	VTE prophylaxis.	The number of patients who received VTE prophylaxis or have documentation why no VTE prophylaxis was given.
VTE 2	NQF 0372	Intensive care unit VTE prophylaxis.	The number of patients who received VTE prophylaxis or have documentation why no VTE prophylaxis was given the day of or the day after the initial admission or transfer to the intensive care unit or surgery end date for surgeries that start the day of or the day after ICU admission or transfer.
VTE 3	NQF 0373	VTE patients with anticoagulant overlap therapy.	Number of patients with diagnosed VTE who received an overlap of anticoagulation and warfarin therapy.
VTE 4	Not applicable	VTE patients receiving unfractionated heparin with dosages/platelet count monitoring by protocol or nomogram.	Number of patients diagnosed with confirmed VTE who received intravenous (IV) UFH therapy dosages AND had their platelet counts monitored using defined parameters such as a nomogram or protocol.
VTE 5	Not applicable	VTE warfarin therapy discharge instructions.	Number of patients diagnosed with confirmed VTE that are discharged to home, home care, court/law enforcement or home on hospice care on warfarin with written discharge instructions that address all four criteria: compliance issues, dietary advice, follow-up monitoring, and information about the potential for adverse drug reactions/interactions.

(continued on next page)

TJC Identifier	NQF Identifier	Description	Measurement
Table 2 *(continued)*			
VTE 6	Not applicable	Hospital acquired potentially-preventable VTE.	Number of patients diagnosed with confirmed VTE during hospitalization (not present at admission) who did not receive VTE prophylaxis between hospital admission and the day before the VTE diagnostic testing order date.
STK 1	NQF 0434	VTE prophylaxis.	Ischemic and hemorrhagic stroke patients who received VTE prophylaxis or have documentation why no VTE prophylaxis was given on the day of or the day after hospital admission.
STK 2	NQF 0435	Discharged on antithrombotic therapy.	Ischemic stroke patients prescribed antithrombotic therapy at hospital discharge.
STK 3	NQF 0436	Anticoagulation therapy for atrial fibrillation/flutter	Ischemic stroke patients with atrial fibrillation/flutter who are prescribed anticoagulation at discharge

Abbreviation: NQF, national quality forum.

chart-abstracted measures, electronic Clinical Quality Measure (CQM), or a combination of both. This information flows to TJC and CMS and ultimately should return to practicing clinicians as a method of identifying areas of practice improvement (**Fig. 2**). Hospital participation in the CMS IQR Program has increased to greater than 99% of all acute care hospitals since CMS introduced the financial penalty.[13,14] Hospitals that do not comply with these reporting standards are subject to loss of TJC accreditation and CMS penalties. For fiscal year 2016, CMS has altered the payment structure.[15] Hospitals that participate in the IQR Program and are submitting electronic CQM records will receive a 0.9% increase in operating payment rates. In addition, the market basket rate (an adjustment for inflation of costs incurred by hospitals during the provision of patient care) will be 2.4%. However, the market basket rate will be 25% lower (1.8%) for hospitals that are noncompliant with CMS reporting standards.

TARGETED PERFORMANCE STANDARDS
Stroke Management Standards

The American Stroke Association, American Heart Association, Agency for Health Quality and Research (AHRQ), American Speech-Language-Hearing Association, Centers for Disease Control and Prevention, and TJC collectively crafted 17 performance standards with a goal of improving care quality, ensuring accountability, and providing information to the public.[16] Within the standards, several measures specifically address VTE prevention and safe anticoagulant use (see **Table 2**). Surveillance research has suggested that similar practice standards improve performance

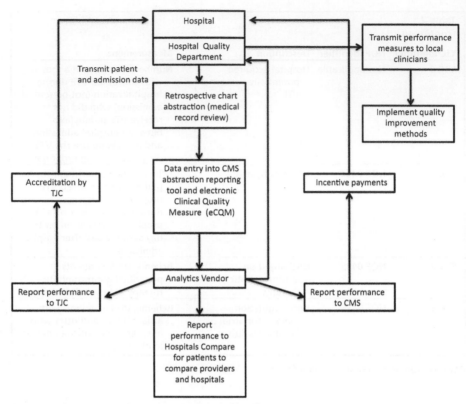

Fig. 2. Performance and outcome measure data flow.

measure adherence, early anticoagulant use, and prescription at discharge.[17] A recent review of stroke care showed a significant improvement in quality of care metrics.[18] Designated primary stroke centers have shown improved compliance with performance measures but with room for further improvement.[19] However, a recent review evaluating compliance with stroke standards suggests patient outcome data are limited.

Stroke severity varies considerably among patients and is a key determinant of patient outcomes despite established evidence-based guidelines and endorsed standards. The value of performance standards and measurements require more study and therefore clinicians should be prepared to further evaluate the relationships between quality metrics and patient outcomes.[20]

SURGICAL CARE IMPROVEMENT PROJECTS

CMS, after collaboration with other government agencies, professional organizations, and regulatory agencies, implemented the Surgical Care Improvement Project (SCIP). The project included a goal of reducing VTE-related events by 25% in patients undergoing surgical procedures.[21] Despite evidence-based guidelines for VTE prevention strategies, VTE prophylaxis is often underused.[22] SCIP introduced two methods for improving VTE prophylaxis utilization. The first measure assessed whether VTE prophylaxis was ordered and the second measured whether prophylaxis was received, both within 24 hours after surgical procedure (see **Table 2**).[23] The CMS "pay for performance" structure prompted hospitals to implement the SCIP measures and comply with TJC surveys and the National Quality Forum–endorsed measures.[8,24] Similar to stroke measures, the SCIP VTE prophylaxis adherence rates have improved. However, there still are limited data demonstrating that adherence reduces VTE event rates.[24–26]

The actual incidence of postoperative VTE, the optimal duration for observation, and the level of surveillance applied to detect events remains controvesial.[25–28] The in-hospital rates of VTE in patients receiving appropriate thromboprophylaxis after hip and knee arthroplasty were estimated recently at approximately 0.5% and 1% of patients, respectively.[25] The authors have proposed using these rates as an indicator for safety and quality. SCIP VTE events are based on the application of International Classification of Diseases, Ninth Edition, Clinical Modification (ICD-9-CM) hospital discharge codes. The accuracy of this methodology has been challenged.[26] Furthermore, the period of postoperative VTE risk extends well beyond hospitalization in hip (10–12 weeks) and knee arthroplasty (4–6 weeks).[27] Three-month VTE incidence rates reflect the longer period of VTE risk and may be a more appropriate observational period for quality improvement measures. A recent study that evaluated the association of adherence to SCIP thromboprophylaxis protocols and VTE rates found that hospitals that consistently adhered to VTE reduction protocols had higher rates of VTE, primarily because of increased surveillance and imaging use.[28]

Although interhospital comparisons may be inappropriate alternative options for VTE monitoring, standards for when to image, screening all patients during hospitalization, and development of new, more accurate VTE measures may not be feasible.[29] The existing measures still offer important information for evaluating performance and practices with a single facility. Data collection, identifying events, and segregating higher risk patient populations afford an opportunity for improvement-targeted VTE prevention interventions. These data may help identify low-risk patients for whom prophylaxis offers no benefit. It may also identify high-risk patients with breakthrough thrombosis despite seemingly adequate prophylaxis who may require combination preventive strategies.

POINT SCORING SYSTEMS
Hospital Acquired Conditions Reduction Program

HHS is required to identify high-cost, high-volume conditions that result in a higher hospital payment, but could have been prevented by the application of evidence-based guidelines.[30] CMS developed a list of hospital-acquired conditions (HACs) that are considered preventable events if not present on admission. Included was deep vein thrombosis (DVT) or pulmonary embolism (PE) following total hip or knee replacement. Although a patient's initial stay was eligible for CMS reimbursement, hospitals no longer received reimbursement for the additional expenses associated with hospital-acquired DVT or PE.[31] In 2009, the Patient Protection and Affordable Care Act established the HAC Reduction Program, which eliminated CMS payments for HACs and introduced a point scoring system to provide an incentive for hospitals to reduce these events. A total HAC point score (**Fig. 3**) is calculated for each hospital based on performance on AHRQ Patient Safety Indicators (PSI). Included in the point score is the incidence of postoperative DVT and PE. CMS payments are then determined based on a hospital's total HAC point score and their comparison with the HAC score of other hospitals. HAC point scores are publicly available on the Hospital Compare Web site. In 2015, approximately 724 hospitals nationwide received a 1% reduction (penalty) in Medicare payments for poor HAC-related outcomes.

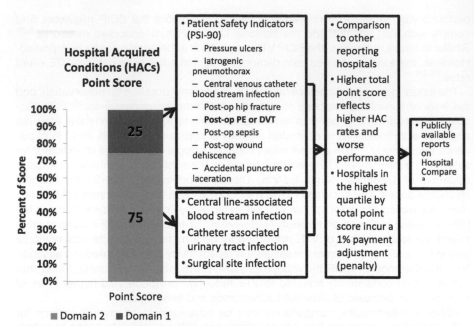

Fig. 3. Hospital-acquired conditions point scoring and hospital payments. [a] https://www.medicare.gov/hospitalcompare/search.html.

HHS has recently reported the improvement in patient outcomes from the program, estimating 50,000 deaths averted and $12 billion in spending avoided over the time period of 2010 to 2013.[32] Postoperative VTE was reduced from 28,000 events in 2010 to 23,000 events in 2013. This 18% reduction in events was estimated to have avoid 520 deaths and saved the US health care system approximately $40 million. HHS attributed the success to payment policies, public reporting of hospital performance, and the assistance from nonprofit organizations.

Hospital Consumer Assessment of Healthcare Providers and Systems and the Five Star Quality Rating System

CMS established the Hospital Consumer Assessment of Healthcare Providers and Systems (HCAHPS) rating to give consumers easily accessible information on the patient experience. The system uses an 11-measure patient survey tool (**Table 3**) to generate a final score.[33] The score is intended to help patients compare health care providers and systems. Patients treated on anticoagulation therapy have been shown to have increased satisfaction with patient education and care coordination when care is directed by an anticoagulation management service. Because warfarin patient and family education is mandated by TJC standards, there is an opportunity to impact HCAHPS scores surrounding the elements patient satisfaction and quality of care.[34] The HCAHPS score is a component of the CMS Value Based Purchasing Program, which effects Medicare reimbursement.[35] The CMS new Overall Hospital Quality Star Rating System (OHQSRS) is designed to make comparative health care information more accessible to patients. OHQSRS incorporates a hospital's IQR performance and PSI measures, and Outpatient Quality Reporting program data (**Fig. 4**). The rating consolidates 75 measures into a single, easy to interpret five star rating system that will be available on the CMS Hospital Compare Web site. Consumers and patients

Table 3
HCAHPS and STAR ratings

HCAHPS Measures	Eleven HCAHPS Measure Star Rating	Nine Star Ratings Used in HCAPHS	Nine-Measure Average		Star Rating
Communication with RNs	5	5	(5 + 4 + 4 + 3	4	
Communications with MDs	4	4	+ 5 + 4 + 4 + 5 + 3.5)/		
Responsiveness of hospital staff	4	4	9 = 4.17		
Pain management	3	3			
Communication about medicines	5	5			
Discharge information	4	4		Stars	Range
Care transitions	4	4		1	1–1.49
Cleanliness	5	(5 + 5)/2 = 5		2	1.5–2.49
Quietness	5			3	2.5–3.49
Overall rating	3	(3 + 4)/2 = 3.5		4	3.5–4.49
Recommend the hospital	4			5	4.5–5

in the past have stated that most past rating systems are difficult to interpret. The system measures include outcomes (mortality, readmissions, safety), process of care delivery (timeliness, effectiveness), patient experience, and efficiency.[36] The implementation of OHQSRS has been delayed until July 2016 to allow CMS additional time to communicate to providers and make any final methodology adjustments.[37]

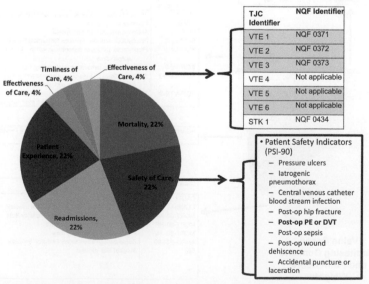

Fig. 4. Components of the stars scoring methodology. NQF, national quality forum.

Value Based Purchasing

In 2011 CMS launched the Hospital Value-Based Purchasing (VBP) program, a new initiative designed to adjust reimbursement based on quality measurements further emphasizing the transition from "pay for reporting" to" pay for performance." CMS calculates a total performance score that is based on four weighted domains of care (**Fig. 5**). Quality measurements from CMS's IQR program (SCIP-VTE 1, SCIP-VTE 2), HCAHPS score, and the AHRQ Patient PSI list are included as part of the initial measures for the new VBP program.[35] Individual measures may be added, changed, or retired over time. For example, some clinical process measures may "top out" as variability among hospitals diminishes and performance approaches 100%. Using the final calculated VBP score Medicare payments or penalties are given to promote a higher quality of care.[38]

ELECTRONIC HEALTH RECORD MEANINGFUL USE

The Health Information Technology for Economic and Clinical Health Act (2009) provides HHS with the authority to establish programs that promote the use of information technology. CMS has provided financial incentives to promote the "meaningful use" of electronic health records (EHR).[39] Eligible professionals and hospitals may implement EHR and attain CMS-established goals according to a three-stage plan. Stage 1 mandates data capture and information sharing, stage 2 requires use of advanced clinical processes, and stage 3 focuses on improved health outcomes. Providers and hospitals must meet thresholds for certain objectives within each stage of the plan. Recently CMS made adjustments to the requirements for stages 2 and 3 (**Table 4**).[40] Embedded in the Clinical Decision Support requirements are CQMs. These mandated interventions are the same quality measures (VTE-1, VTE-2, VTE-3, VTE-4, VTE-5, STK-2, STK-3, STK-4, STK-5, and so forth) that are part of the IQR Program. Penalties exist for those who fail to incorporate meaningful use EHR. For example, the Medicare

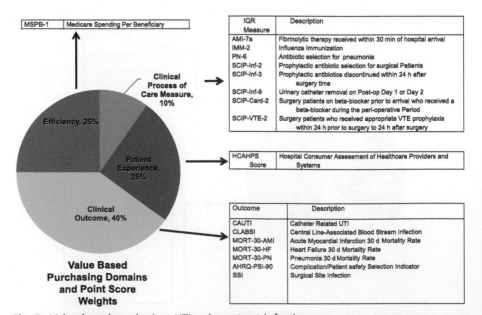

Fig. 5. Value-based purchasing. UTI, urinary tract infection.

Table 4
Electronic health records meaningful use requirements for stage 2 and stage 3

Objective	Modified Stage 2 and Stage 3 Requirements
Protect Patient Health Information	Conduct the security risk analysis with installation/update EHR Technology.
Electronic Prescribing (eRx)	10% to >80% of all hospital discharge RXs are queried for drug formulary status & transmitted electronically.
Clinical Decision Support	Measure 1: Implement 5 clinical decision support interventions related to >4 or more CQMs at a relevant point in patient care. Measure 2: Implement drug-drug and drug-allergy interaction checks.
Computerized Provider Order Entry	Must meet all three measures in order to meet this objective: Measure 1: >60% to >80% of medication orders, Measure 2: >30% to >60% of laboratory orders, Measure 3: >30% to >60% of diagnostic imaging orders are recorded using CPOE.
Health Information Exchange	Measure 1: Transitions of care and referrals have; (1) a summary of care record using CEHRT; and (2) electronic exchanges the summary of care record. Measure 2: >10% to >40% of transitions or referrals incorporates an electronic summary of care from another provider's EHR system. Measure 3: >80% of transitions or referrals the provider performs a clinical information reconciliation. For Medication, Medication allergy, and Current Problem list.
Patient-specific education resources	>10% of all unique patients admitted to the hospital or CAH inpatient or emergency department are provided patient specific education resources as defined by CEHRT.
Medication Reconciliation	The hospital or CAH performs medication reconciliation for >50% of transition of care on admission to inpatient or emergency department.
Patient Electronic Access	Measure 1: 50% to >80% of patients can view online, download, and transmit their health information within 24 hours of its availability to the provider. Measure 2: Use CEHRT to identify patient-specific educational resources and provide electronic access to those materials to >35% of patients.
Coordination of Care	Must meet 2 of 3 measures to meet the objective: Measure 1: >25% of patients actively engage with the EHR made accessible by the provider. Measure 2: >35% of all patients received or responded to a secure message as sent using the electronic messaging function of CEHRT Measure 3: Patient-generated health data or data from a non-clinical setting is incorporated into the certified EHR technology for >15% of all patients
Public Health Reporting	Providers must meet 2 of 3 measures: Immunization Registry Reporting through Public Health Agency Syndromic Surveillance Reporting Registry Reporting Clinical Data Registry Reporting.

Abbreviations: CAH, critical access hospital; CEHRT, certified electronic health record technology; CPOE, computer physician order entry; CQM, clinical quality measures; EHR, electronic health records.

physician fee schedule is adjusted downward by 1% each year beginning in 2015 up to a maximum of 5% in 2020 for eligible professionals who are not meaningful EHR users. For hospitals, the Inpatient Prospective Payment System rate is adjusted downward by 25% in 2015, 50% in 2016 and 75% in 2017 and beyond. Therefore, data submitted to CMS for incentive payment consideration should include CQMs derived from meaningfully used EHRs.

THE NATIONAL ACTION PLAN FOR ADVERSE DRUG EVENT PREVENTION

HHS recently created the National Action Plan for Adverse Drug Event Prevention (ADE Action Plan) through the alignment and efforts of numerous federal health care agencies. This effort is intended to identify common, preventable ADEs with the goal of reducing patient harm.[7] Anticoagulants are one of the three initial drug classes that are high-priority targets. The Plan recommends a four-pronged approach (surveillance, prevention, incentive and oversight, and research) with action steps incorporated into each strategy (**Fig. 6**).

The Plan includes standardizing event definitions (anticoagulant-associated bleeding, thrombosis events), integrating EHR (hospital, laboratory, pharmacy), and outcomes data. The Plan focuses on incorporating current evidence-based guidelines, protocols, and dosing algorithms for anticoagulant use into daily practice.[41] It incorporates anticoagulation best practices (patient self-management, patient and family engagement, communication, and care coordination) from a variety of organizations (TJC, the Institute for Safe Medication Practices, National Quality Forum, and the Anticoagulation Forum) for inpatient and outpatient settings (**Table 5**).[42–45] It recommends the formation of anticoagulant stewardship programs and patient enrollment in anticoagulation clinics, which have shown to improve anticoagulation management and reduce health care costs.[46–50]

The Plan is expected to use regulatory tactics to incentivize practice changes. These include CMS performance measures, TJC surveys for compliance and compulsory reporting, and payment adjustments with either incentives or penalties.

Health information technology and its exchange infrastructure are important components of the Plan. The Plan has identified recognized exiting clinical guidelines and anticoagulation quality measures that have been nationally endorsed. Several of these measures are expected to be incorporated into the stage 3 EHR meaningful use requirements with a goal of impacting outcomes through decision support.

POSTMARKETING SURVEILLANCE

In 2008, HHS and the Food and Drug Administration (FDA) announced the Sentinel Initiative, a program designed to enhance the existing postmarketing safety system into an active postmarketing safety and performance monitoring system.[51,52] The Mini-Sentinel program integrates current FDA surveillance capabilities with those of multiple partners. The partners provide technical and methodologic support. Health care organizations supply information for millions of patients. A data coordinating center accesses automated health care data systems (eg, EHR systems, administrative claims databases, pharmacy dispensing, registries) using existing standardized coding (ICD-9-CM, Healthcare Common Procedure codes, Current Procedural Terminology codes, National Drug Code). This allows for rapid and secure queries of disparate but standardized data sources for relevant product use and safety outcomes. In the past these queries were limited to one health care system or one claims database.

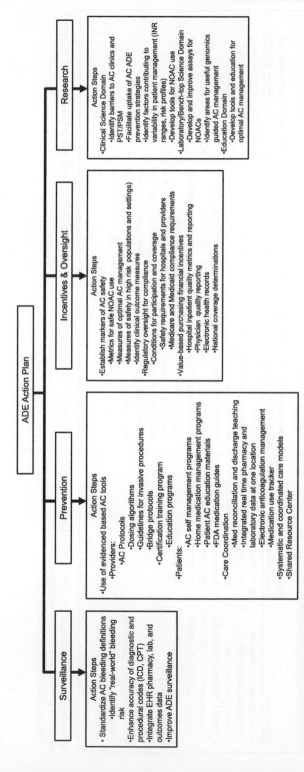

Fig. 6. National Adverse Event Action Plan for reducing harm with anticoagulants. AC, anticoagulants; ADE adverse drug event; CPT, current procedural terminology; EHR, electronic health record; FDA, food and drug administration; ICD international classification of disease; INR, international normalized ratio; NOAC, novel oral anticoagulant; TTR, time within therapeutic range.

Table 5
Adverse drug event action plan best practices

Safer Care	Patient and Family Engagement	Promotion of Best Practices Within Communities	Science-Driven Prevention and Treatment	Effective Communication and Coordination of Care
• Continuously improve provider knowledge through education • Use of evidence-based AC management models (AMS clinics, warfarin PST/PSM) • Address provider concerns surrounding supratherapeutic INRs (falls, bleeding) • Develop NOAC guidelines/algorithms to fill gaps in evidence and provider knowledge	Incorporate anticoagulation-specific patient management into chronic disease education programs and other patient education/health literacy tools	• Promote the adoption of standards of high-quality AC management (eg, Anticoagulation Center of Excellence) • Support sharing of strategies and results from quality-improvement learning initiatives among health care systems and facilities	• Better use NOACs in national health care quality/patient safety measures and national clinical guidelines • Address variability among practice sites • Identify patients at high risk for bleeding events by addressing gaps in guidelines (eg, bleeding score effectiveness in relation to NOACs)	• Improve EHR tools for real-time integrated history-medication-laboratory data • Integrate anticoagulant-specific targets into existing transition of care models

Abbreviations: AC, anticoagulant; AMS, anticoagulation management service; INR, international normalized ratio; NOAC, novel oral anticoagulant; PSM, patent self-management; PST, patient self-treatment. Reduction in AC related ADEs.

The FDA has reported two Drug Safety Communications surrounding dabigatran, representing the completion of three medication use evaluations through the Mini-Sentinel event project.[53,54] The investigators used the previous mentioned strategy to evaluate gastrointestinal hemorrhage (GIH) and intracerebral hemorrhage (ICH) in newly treated patients with dabigatran and warfarin.[55] ICD-9-CM codes were used to identify AF, GIH, and ICH. National Drug Codes were used to identify dabigatran and warfarin treatments. Patients with pre-existing AF and those without any pre-existing conditions were included provided they had a prior 6-month history of health plan and prescription coverage. Bleeding events were counted only if there had been no prior event within the last 183 days of warfarin or dabigatran dispensing. Bleeding events were counted up to 10 days after the treatment period ended. Encounters were limited to inpatient and emergency department visits. Event rates were reported based on days at risk. The results showed the individual incidence rates for GIH (2.0 vs 3.4 events per 100,000 days at risk) and ICH (0.8 vs 2.4 events per 100,000 days at risk) were lower with dabigatran when compared with warfarin. The investigators concluded bleeding rates associated with dabigatran use did not seem to be higher than warfarin.

The FDA continued its ongoing surveillance by completing a follow-up retrospective review of an elderly Medicare patient population initiating dabigatran or warfarin for nonvalvular AF.[56] Investigators used the Mini-Sentinel event system to identify patients through office-based, hospitalization, and drug prescription claims. Patients had to be older than 65 years and enrolled in Medicare for at least 6 months before receiving a prescription for dabigatran or warfarin. AF and the primary outcomes of ischemic stroke, ICH, GIH, and acute myocardial infarction were identified using ICD-9-CM codes. Dabigatran use was associated with a reduced risk of ischemic stroke (hazard ratio, 0.80; 95% confidence interval, 0.67–0.96), ICH (hazard ratio, 0.34; 95% confidence interval, 0.26–0.46), and death (hazard ratio, 0.86; 95% confidence interval, 0.77–0.96) but an increase in GIH (hazard ratio, 1.38; 95% confidence interval, 1.14–1.44). The investigators found their results were similar to those found in the RE-LY trial.

The Mini-Sentinel project is intended to complement clinical trials and existing FDA voluntary reporting programs, such as MedWatch. The Mini-Sentinel Prospective Routine Observational Monitoring Program Tools (PROMPT) is ongoing and will follow a similar methodology, evaluating rivaroxaban and warfarin-treated AF cohorts matched on propensity scores.[57] Clinicians will be faced with becoming familiar with these analyses, translating them into practice change, and building confidence in their evidence-based prescribing patterns.

PRODUCT CONTAMINATION AND PHARMACEUTICAL SUPPLY CHAIN

Identification of contaminated and/or counterfeited imported pharmaceutical products, highlighted by the 2008 heparin crisis, has prompted scrutiny of the FDA in its ability to ensure the safety of imported products.[58,59] The initial response to these tragedies was stricter enforcement by the FDA of its own standards[58] and the introduction of new quality assays, including two screening methods (capillary electrophoresis and proton nuclear magnetic resonance). These processes ensure the quality testing of all heparin products intended for the US market and have been included in the US Pharmacopeia monograph since June 2008.

More recently, Congress passed the FDA Safety and Innovation Act and the Drug Supply Chain Security Act to enhance the ability of the FDA to secure pharmaceuticals.[60,61] The FDA has also implemented the Secure Supply Chain Pilot Program, which is designed to increase inspection of products identified as high-risk for counterfeiting.[61] When fully implemented, the program will allow the FDA to track contaminated or counterfeited products at the individual package level, using unique identifiers throughout the supply chain.

LITIGATION

Serious and fatal anticoagulant-related ADEs lead to product liability and litigation. Dabigatran-related ADEs initially had 21 lawsuits pending in 11 US district courts filed against its manufacturer, Boehringer-Ingelheim.[62] The allegations included lack of proper communication of the bleed to patients and health care providers, and the lack of a reversal agent for bleeding events. In August 2012, the US Judicial Panel on Multidistrict Litigation consolidated all the dabigatran lawsuits into a multidistrict litigation, centralized in Illinois.

In May 2014, Boehringer-Ingelheim agreed to pay $650 million to resolve 2607 cases and settle with 2688 plaintiffs. In agreeing to the multidistrict litigation settlement, Boehringer-Ingelheim denied any wrongdoing. Only individuals who had already filed a case or retained an attorney were eligible to participate. This settlement does not prevent new legal actions against Boehringer-Ingelheim.

Litigation surrounding rivaroxaban is in its early stages but following a similar path.[63] There are 21 actions pending in 10 districts with cases of uncontrollable bleeding, hospitalization, and death coupled with allegations of inadequate warning labels with respect to severe or fatal bleeding, the lack of a reversal agent, and the need for blood monitoring. In December 2014, US Judicial Panel on Multidistrict Litigation consolidated and centralized all nationwide rivaroxaban lawsuits to the Eastern District of Louisiana.[64]

Clinicians can expect to see more litigation for approved anticoagulant agents and patient questions and concerns. Many patients will hear and respond to media advertisements prompting ADE reporting and opportunities for litigation. This highlights the necessity for patient counseling on risks and medication compliance and medical documentation to help avoid adverse outcomes.

SUMMARY

The role of regulatory, legislative, and nonprofit organizations continues to grow in health care. Behind the scene of patient encounters, information on practice patterns, process of care delivery, and outcomes are being collected, submitted, and analyzed by several agencies. Performance measures, practice standards, and point scoring systems are shaping the daily tasks of clinicians and influencing the outcomes of patient treatments. Clinicians should recognize that these organizations work collaboratively and their programs are intertwined, often in a way that alters practice. Most initiatives foster change through reimbursement incentives or penalties.

Many patients require treatment or prevention of thrombosis. Anticoagulants are considered high-risk medications and are routinely the topic of new professional guidelines and new practice standards. The ADE represents the initial step in developing a nationwide, comprehensive set of best practices for anticoagulation management. It outlines the interventions for providing high-quality anticoagulation management and the initial metrics for measuring success. Clinicians should be aware of and embrace programs that attempt to optimize anticoagulant use and ensure patient safety.

There is a heavy emphasis on the use of EHR. With the ability to merge various databases from inpatient and outpatient settings, many organizations have the ability to follow patients longitudinally and monitor their outcomes. Clinicians will be faced with assessing this information, comparing it with results from clinical trials, and deciding whether there is sufficient evidence to make changes in their practice.

With readily available patient information, unintended consequences of drug therapy are open for review, analysis, and possibly litigation directed at the product, the practitioner, or both. Clinicians must be aware of the pitfalls of anticoagulation therapy and make adjustments in their patient selection, prescribing, and risk-benefit information that is transmitted to the patient and family. Clinicians can expect continuous regulatory requirements that impact thrombosis treatment, prevention, and anticoagulant use.

REFERENCES

1. Roger VL, Go AS, Lloyd-Jones DM, et al. Heart disease and stroke statistics-2012 update: a report from the American Heart Association. Circulation 2012;125(1): e2–220.
2. Brown DL, Boden-Albala B, Langa KM, et al. Projected costs of ischemic stroke in the United States. Neurology 2006;67(8):1390–5.
3. Mahan CE, Borrego ME, Woersching AL, et al. Venous thromboembolism: annualised United States models for total, hospital-acquired and preventable costs utilising long-term attack rates. Thromb Haemost 2012;108(2):291–302.
4. Huang W, Goldberg RJ, Anderson FA, et al. Secular trends in occurrence of acute venous thromboembolism: the Worcester VTE study (1985-2009). Am J Med 2014;127(9):829–39.
5. Fanikos J, Stapinski C, Koo S, et al. Medication errors associated with anticoagulant therapy in the hospital. Am J Cardiol 2014;94(4):532–5.
6. Piazza G, Nguyen TN, Cios D, et al. Anticoagulation-associated adverse drug events. Am J Med 2011;124(12):1136–42.
7. US Department of Health and Human Services, Office of Disease Prevention and Health Promotion. National action plan for adverse drug event prevention. Washington, DC: US Department of Health and Human Services; 2014.
8. Mahan CE. Regulatory, policy and quality update for venous thromboembolism and stroke in United States hospitals. Thromb Res 2012;130(4):586–90.
9. Dusetzina SB, Higashi AS, Dorsey ER, et al. Impact of FDA drug risk communications on health care utilization and health behaviors: a systematic review. Med Care 2012;50(6):466–78.
10. Chassin MR, Loeb JM, Schmaltz SP, et al. Accountability measures: using measurements to promote quality improvement. N Engl J Med 2010;363(7):683–8.
11. The Joint Commission. Facts about ORYX for hospitals (National Hospital Quality Measures). 2014. Available at: http://www.jointcommission.org/facts_about_oryx_for_hospitals. Accessed February 5, 2015.
12. The Joint Commission. 2015 flexible ORYX performance measure reporting options. 2014. Available at: http://www.jointcommission.org/assets/1/18/2015_OPTIONS_UPDATED_11-4_15.pdf. Accessed February 5, 2015.
13. Consumer Purchaser Alliance. Fact sheet: Hospital Inpatient Quality Reporting (IQR) Program. 2014. Available at: http://consumerpurchaser.org/files/IQR_FactSheet.pdf. Accessed February 5, 2015.
14. The Centers for Medicare and Medicaid Services. Fact sheets: CMS to improve quality of care during hospital inpatients stays. 2014. Available at: http://www.cms.gov/Newsroom/MediaReleaseDatabase/Fact-sheets/2014-Fact-sheets-items/2014-08-04-2.html. Accessed February 5, 2015.

15. The Joint Commission. Facts about ORYX for Hospitals (National Hospital Quality Measures). The Joint Commission, [Internet]. Available at: https://www.joint commission.org/facts_about_oryx_for_hospitals/. Accessed May 16, 2016.
16. The National Quality Forum. National voluntary consensus standards for stroke prevention and management across the continuum of care: a consensus report. 2010. Available at: http://www.qualityforum.org/Publications/2010/02/National_Voluntary_Consensus_Standards_for_Stroke_Prevention_and_Management_Across_the_Continuum_of_Care.aspx. Accessed December 2, 2014.
17. LaBresh KA, Reeves MJ, Frankel MR, et al. Hospital treatment of patients with ischemic stroke or transient ischemic attack using the "Get With The Guidelines" program. Arch Intern Med 2008;168(4):411–7.
18. Fonarow GC, Reeves MJ, Smith EE, et al. Characteristics, performance measures, and in-hospital outcomes of the first one million stroke and transient ischemic attack admissions in "Get with the Guidelines"-stroke. Circ Cardiovasc Qual Outcomes 2010;3(3):291–302.
19. Johnson AM, Goldstein LB, Bennett P, et al. Compliance with acute stroke care quality measures in hospitals with and without primary stroke center certification: the North Carolina Stroke Care Collaborative. J Am Heart Assoc 2014;3(2): e000423.
20. Parker C, Schwamm LH, Fonarow GC, et al. Stroke quality metrics: systematic reviews of the relationships to patient-centered outcomes and impact of public reporting. Stroke 2012;43(1):155–62.
21. Blatzer D, Hunt D. The surgical infection prevention and surgical care improvement projects: national initiatives to improve outcomes for patients having surgery. Clin Infect Dis 2006;43:322–30.
22. Stratton MA, Anderson FA, Bussey HI, et al. Prevention of venous thromboembolism: adherence to the 1995 American College of Chest Physicians consensus guidelines for surgical patients. Arch Intern Med 2000;160(3):334–40.
23. Altom LK, Deierhoi RJ, Grams J, et al. Association between Surgical Care Improvement Program venous thromboembolism measures and postoperative events. Am J Surg 2012;204(5):591–7.
24. Hawn MT, Itani KM, Gray SH, et al. Association of timely administration of prophylactic antibiotics for major surgical procedures and surgical site infection. J Am Coll Surg 2008;206(5):814–9 [discussion: 819–21].
25. Januel JM, Chen G, Ruffieux C, et al. Symptomatic in-hospital deep vein thrombosis and pulmonary embolism following hip and knee arthroplasty among patients receiving recommended prophylaxis: a systematic review. JAMA 2012; 307(3):294–303.
26. White RH, Sadeghi B, Tancredi DJ, et al. How valid is the ICD-9-CM based AHRQ patient safety indicator for postoperative venous thromboembolism? Med Care 2009;47(12):1237–43.
27. Heit JA. Estimating the incidence of symptomatic postoperative venous thromboembolism: the importance of perspective. JAMA 2012;307(3):306–7.
28. Bilimoria KY, Chung J, Ju MH. Evaluation of surveillance bias and the validity of the venous thromboembolism quality measure. JAMA 2013;310(14):1482–9.
29. Yang AD, Bilimoria KY. Accurately measuring hospital venous thromboembolism prevention efforts. JAMA 2016;35:2113–4.
30. US Department of Health and Human Services, Centers for Medicare and Medicaid Services. CMS to improve quality of care during hospital inpatient stays [Internet]. 2014. Available at: http://www.cms.gov/Newsroom/MediaReleaseDatabase/Factsheets/2014-Fact-sheets-items/2014-08-04-2.html. Accessed December 4, 2014.

31. Centers for Medicare and Medicaid Services. Hospital-acquired conditions (present on admission indicator). Available at: http://www.cms.gov/Medicare/Medicare-Fee-for-Service-Payment/HospitalAcqCond/Downloads/FY_2013_Final_HACsCodeList.pdf. Accessed December 2, 2014.

32. US Department of Health and Human Services. Interim update on 2013 annual hospital-acquired condition rate and estimates of cost savings and deaths averted from 2010 to 2013. 2014. Available at: http://www.ahrq.gov/professionals/quality-patient-safety/pfp/interimhacrate2013.pdf. Accessed December 2, 2014.

33. HCAPHS star rating technical notes. HCAHPS Online. CMS, [Internet]. Available at: http://www.hcahpsonline.org/Files/July_2016_Star%20Ratings_Tech%20Notes.pdf. Accessed May 16, 2016.

34. Makowski CT, Jennings DL, Nemerovski CW, et al. The impact of pharmacist directed patient education and anticoagulant care coordination on patient safety. Ann Pharmacother 2013;47:805–10.

35. Hospital Value-Based Purchasing. Center for Medicare and Medicaid Services. Department of Health and Human Services, [Internet]. Available at: https://www.cms.gov/Outreach-and-Education/Medicare-Learning-Network-MLN/MLNProducts/downloads/Hospital_VBPurchasing_Fact_Sheet_ICN907664.pdf. Accessed May 16, 2016.

36. Yale New Haven Health Center for outcomes research and evaluation hospital quality star ratings on hospital compare. Dry run, methodology of Overall Hospital Quality Star Ratings. [Internet]. 2015. Available at: http://essentialhospitals.org/wp-content/uploads/2015/07/OvrHosQualStrRtgsDryRnMeth2015.pdf. Accessed May 19, 2016.

37. Centers for Medicare and Medicaid Services. July 2016 Overall Star Rating HSR Guide (HUG). [Internet]. 2016. Available at: https://www.qualitynet.org/dcs/ContentServer?c=Page&pagename=QnetPublic%2FPage%2FQnetTier2&cid=1228775183434. Accessed May 19, 2016.

38. Center for Medicare and Medicaid Services. Hospital acquired condition reduction program fiscal year 2016 fact sheet. 2016. Available at: https://www.qualitynet.org/dcs/BlobServer?blobkey=id&blobnocache=true&blobwhere=1228890507799&blobheader=multipart%2Foctet-stream&blobheadername1=Content-Disposition&blobheadervalue1=attachment%3Bfilename%3DFY_2016_HACRP_FactSheet.pdf&blobcol=urldata&blobtable=MungoBlobs. Accessed May 17, 2016.

39. The Centers for Medicare and Medicaid Services. 2014 definition of stage 1 of meaningful use. 2014. Available at: http://www.cms.gov/Regulations-and-Guidance/Legislation/EHRIncentivePrograms/Meaningful_Use.html. Accessed February 5, 2015.

40. The Federal Register. Medicare and Medicaid Programs; Electronic Health Record Incentive Program-Stage 3 and modifications to meaningful use in 2015 through 2017. Available at: https://www.federalregister.gov/articles/2015/10/16/2015-25595/medicare-and-medicaid-programs-electronic-health-record-incentive-program-stage-3-and-modifications#h-186. Accessed May 1, 2016.

41. Holbrook A, Schulman S, Witt DM, et al. Evidence-based management of anticoagulant therapy: antithrombotic therapy and prevention of thrombosis, 9th ed: American College of Chest Physicians Evidence-Based Clinical Practice Guidelines. Chest 2012;141(2 Suppl):e152S–84S.

42. The Joint Commission. 2014 Hospital National Patient Safety Goals. [Internet]. 2014. Available at: http://jointcomission.org/assets/1/6/2014_HAFP_NPSG_E.pdf. Accessed December 4, 2014.

43. Institute for Safe Medication Practices. Organizations release new tools for reducing medication errors. 2002. Available at: http://ismp.org/tools/pathways.asp. Accessed December 4, 2014.

44. The National Quality Forum. Measures, reports & tools. 2013. Available at: http://www.qualityforum.org/measures_reports_tools.aspx. Accessed December 4, 2014.

45. Nutescu EA, Wittkowsky AK, Burnett A, et al. Delivery of optimized inpatient anticoagulation therapy: consensus statement from the anticoagulation forum. Ann Pharmacother 2013;47(5):714–24.

46. Rudd KM, Dier JG. Comparison of two different models of anticoagulation management services with usual medical care. Pharmacotherapy 2010;30(4): 330–8.

47. Witt DM, Humphries TL. A retrospective evaluation of the management of excessive anticoagulation in an established clinical pharmacy anticoagulation service compared to traditional care. J Thromb Thrombolysis 2003;15(2): 113–8.

48. Bungard TJ, Gardner L, Archer SL, et al. Evaluation of a pharmacist-managed anticoagulation clinic: improving patient care. Open Med 2009;3(1):e16–21.

49. Ansell JE, Hughes R. Evolving models of warfarin management: anticoagulation clinics, patient self-monitoring, and patient self-management. Am Heart J 1996; 132(5):1095–100.

50. Gray DR, Garabedian-Ruffalo SM, Chretien SD. Cost-justification of a clinical pharmacist-managed anticoagulation clinic. Ann Pharmacother 2007;41(3): 496–501.

51. Behrman RE, Benner JS, Brown JS, et al. Developing the Sentinel System: a national resource for evidence development. N Engl J Med 2011;364(6):498–9.

52. Psaty BM, Breckenridge AM. Mini-Sentinel and regulatory science: big data rendered fit and functional. N Engl J Med 2014;370(23):2165–7.

53. Institute for Safe Medication Practices. Monitoring MedWatch reports: signals for two newly approved drugs and 2010 annual summary. Horsham, PA: QuarterWatch; 2010.

54. Institute for Safe Medication Practices. Signals for dabigatran and metoclopramide. Horsham, PA: QuarterWatch; 2012.

55. Mini-Sentinel. Health outcomes among individuals exposed to medical product details: dabigatran, warfarin & GI bleed, intracerebral hemorrhage [Internet]. 2013. Available at: http://www.mini-sentinel.org/work_products/Assessments/Mini-Sentinel_Modular-Program-Report_MSY3_MPR41_Dabigatran-Warfarin-GIH-ICH_Part-1.pdf. Accessed December 2, 2014.

56. Mini-Sentinel. Health outcomes among individuals exposed to medical product details: dabigatran, warfarin & GI bleed, intracerebral hemorrhage. 2013. Available at: http://www.mini-sentinel.org/work_products/Assessments/Mini-Sentinel_Modular-Program-Report_MSY3_MPR41_Dabigatran-Warfarin-GIH-ICH_Part-2.pdf. Accessed December 2, 2014.

57. Mini-Sentinel. Prospective Routine Observational Monitoring Program Tools (PROMPT): Rivaroxaban Surveillance Plan v2.0 [Internet]. 2013. Available at: http://www.mini-sentinel.org/work_products/Assessments/Mini-Sentinel_PROMPT_Rivaroxaban-Surveillance-Plan.pdf. Accessed December 1, 2014.

58. Rosaia L. Heparin crisis 2008: a tipping point for increased FDA enforcement in the pharma sector? Food Drug Law J 2010;65(3):489–501.

59. Barlas S. FDA starts new light-touch inspections for some imports. P T 2014; 39(6):384–5.

60. US Department of Health and Human Services, Food and Drug Administration. Food and Drug Administration Safety and Innovation Act. 2014.
61. US Department of Health and Human Services, Food and Drug Administration. Drug Supply Chain Security Act. 2014. Available at: http://www.fda.gov/Drugs/DrugSafety/DrugIntegrityandSupplyChainSecurity/DrugSupplyChainSecurityAct/. Accessed December 4, 2014.
62. United States Judicial Panel on Multistate Legislation. Pradaxa (dabigatran etexilate) products liability litigation. MDL 2385, Document 106.
63. United States Judicial Panel on Multistate Legislation. Xarelto (rivaroxaban) products liability litigation MDL 2592, Document 122.
64. Goldhirsch, K. "Xarelto MDL judge sets limits on joint complaint filings". Legal Examiner. [Internet]. Available at: http://newyork.legalexaminer.com/defective-dangerous-products/xarelto-mdl-judge-sets-limits-on-joint-complaint-filings/. Accessed May 16, 2016.

Index

Note: Page numbers of article titles are in **boldface** type.

A

Activated partial thromboplastin time (aPTT), coagulation testing in patients on direct oral
   anticoagulants, 997–1000
      apixaban, 999
      dabigatran, 998
      edoxaban, 999–1000
      rivaroxaban, 998–999
Adverse drug events, litigation related to, 1130
Adverse events, reversal agents for direct oral anticoagulants, **1085–1098**
Andexanet alpha, for reversal of oral direct anticoagulants, 1031, 1091–1093
Animal models, of thrombosis, 1103–1104
Anticoagulants, direct oral, 987–1135
   after joint replacement surgery, **1007–1018**
      efficacy of, 1014
      Factor Xa inhibitors, history of, 1010–1011
      safety of, 1014–1015
      summary of trials to prevent DVT and PE, 1011–1014
   monitoring effect of, **995–1006**
      assessing reversal of, 1003
      diagnostic options, 997–1002
         coagulation testing, 997
         global assays, 1001
         liquid chromatography/tandem mass spectrometry methodology, 1000
         Russell viper venom time, 1001
         screening coagulation tests (PT and aPTT), 997–1000
         testing specific for measurement of direct thrombin inhibitory activity, 1000–1001
      levels of, and clinical outcomes, 1002
      limitations of assays, 1002–1003
   non-vitamin K antagonist, in atrial fibrillation, **1019–1034**
      apixaban, 1026–1027
      background, 1019–1022
         definition and epidemiology of atrial fibrillation, 1019–1021
         warfarin efficacy, safety, and limitations, 1021–1022
      dabigatran, 1022–1023
      edoxaban, 1027
      rivaroxaban, 1023–1026
      specific patient scenarios and populations, 1027–1031
         cardioversion, 1028
         chronic kidney disease, 1028–1029
         managing bleeding, 1030
         measuring anticoagulation, 1029–1030
         mechanical heart valves, 1027–1028

Anticoagulants (*continued*)
    reversal agents, 1030–1031
  perioperative management of, **1073–1084**
    with high thrombotic risk patient, 1076–1077
    in a low bleed risk procedure, 1077–1079
    in a minimal bleed risk procedure, 1074–1076
    in urgent surgery, 1079–1081
  regulatory impact on use of, **1115–1135**
    electronic health record meaningful use, 1124–1126
    litigation, 1130
    National Action Plan for Adverse Drug Event Prevention, 1126
    organization interactions and performance measures, 1116–1119
    point scoring systems, 1121–1124
      Hospital Acquired Conditions Reduction Program, 1121–1122
      Hospital Consumer Assessment of Healthcare Providers and Systems, 1122–1123
      Value-Based Purchasing, 1124
    postmarketing surveillance, 1126–1129
    product contamination and pharmaceutical supply chain, 1129–1130
    surgical care improvement projects, 1120–1121
    targeted performance standards, 1119–1120
      stroke management standards, 1119–1120
  reversal agents for, **1085–1098**
    attributes of, 1086
    current state of, 1088–1090
    future of, 1094
    specific agents for, 1090–1094
      andexanet alpha, 1091–1093
      ciraparantag, 1093–1094
      idarucizumab, 1090–1091
    for vitamin K antagonists, 1086–1088
    when are they needed, 1086
  for treatment of venous thromboembolism, **1035–1051**
    for acute phase of treatment, 1038–1039
    for extended treatment, 1039–1041
    pharmacologic properties of, 1036–1037
    in routine clinical practice, 1046
    in special populations, 1041–1046
    summary of evidence, 1046–1047
  use in special populations, **1053–1071**
    elderly patients over 75 years of age, 1058–1062
    patients at extremes of body weight, 1054–1058
    patients known to have thrombophilia other than cancer, 1066–1067
    patients with cancer, 1066
    patients with moderate or severe renal impairment, 1062–1065
Antidotes. *See* Reversal agents.
Antisense oligonucleotides, reduction of Factor XI levels induced by, 1107–1108
Antithrombins, pharmacology of, in treatment of VTE, 1036–1037
Antithrombotic therapy, direct oral anticoagulants, 987–1135
    after joint replacement surgery, **1007–1018**
    monitoring effect of, **995–1006**

non-vitamin K antagonist, in atrial fibrillation, **1019–1034**
   perioperative management of, **1073–1084**
   regulatory impact on use of, **1115–1135**
   reversal agents for, **1085–1098**
   for treatment of venous thromboembolism, **1035–1051**
   use in special populations, **1053–1071**
  history of, **987–993**
   aspirin use as, 991–992
   discovery of heparin, 988–990
   discovery of the vitamin K antagonists, 990
  intrinsic pathway of coagulation as target for, **1085–1098**
   in models of blood coagulation, 1100–1103
    cascade-waterfall model of thrombin generation, 1100–1101
    kallikrein-kinin system and contact activation, 1103
    tissue factor-initiated thrombin generation and role of Factor XI, 1101
   thrombosis and, 1103–1105
    animal models, 1103–1104
    Factor IX and VIII thrombosis in humans, 1104
    Factor XI thrombosis in humans, 1104–1105
    intrinsic pathway in humans, 1105
    kallikrein-kinin system in humans, 1105
   trials of agents targeting, 1105–1108
    antisense-induced reduction of Factor XI levels, 1107–1108
    Factor IXa inhibitors, 1105–1106
    targeting the kallikrein-kinin system, 1108
Apixaban, for atrial fibrillation, 1026–1027
  monitoring effects of, 999
  reversal of, with andexanet alpha, 1091–1093
  trials comparing oral dosing vs enoxaparin after joint replacement surgery, 1012–1014
Aspirin, utility as an antithrombotic agent, 991–992
Atrial fibrillation, non-vitamin K antagonist of coagulants in, **1019–1034**
   apixaban, 1026–1027
   background, 1019–1022
    definition and epidemiology of, 1019–1021
    warfarin efficacy, safety, and limitations, 1021–1022
   dabigatran, 1022–1023
   edoxaban, 1027
   rivaroxaban, 1023–1026
   specific patient scenarios and populations, 1027–1031
    cardioversion, 1028
    chronic kidney disease, 1028–1029
    managing bleeding, 1030
    measuring anticoagulation, 1029–1030
    mechanical heart valves, 1027–1028
    reversal agents, 1030–1031

B

Bleeding, management of, in patients on oral direct anticoagulants, 1030
  in patients on direct oral anticoagulants, reversal agents for, 1030, **1085–1098**
Body weight, use of direct oral anticoagulants in patients with extremes of, 1054–1058

C

Cancer, use of direct oral anticoagulants in patients with, 1066
Cardioversion, use of direct oral anticoagulants in patients after, 1028–1029
Cascade-waterfall model, of thrombin generation, 1100–1101, 1102
Cisparantag, for reversal of direct oral anticoagulants, 1093–1094
Coagulation, intrinsic pathway of, as target for antithrombotic therapy, **1085–1098**
    in models of blood coagulation, 1100–1103
        cascade-waterfall model of thrombin generation, 1100–1101
        kallikrein-kinin system and contact activation, 1103
        tissue factor-initiated thrombin generation and role of Factor XI, 1101
    thrombosis and, 1103–1105
        animal models, 1103–1104
        Factor IX and VIII thrombosis in humans, 1104
        Factor XI thrombosis in humans, 1104–1105
        intrinsic pathway in humans, 1105
        kallikrein-kinin system in humans, 1105
    trials of agents targeting, 1105–1108
        antisense-induced reduction of Factor XI levels, 1107–1108
        Factor IXa inhibitors, 1105–1106
        targeting the kallikrein-kinin system, 1108
Coagulation testing, in patients on direct oral anticoagulants, **995–1006**
Contact activation, and kallikrein-kinin system, role in thrombin generation, 1103

D

Dabigatran, for atrial fibrillation, 1022–1023
    monitoring effects of, 998
    reversal of, with idarucizumab, 1090–1091
Deep vein thrombosis (DVT), trials of regulation of coagulation in joint replacement surgery
    to prevent, 1011–1012
        efficacy of, 1014
        safety of, 1014–1015
    use of direct oral anticoagulants for treatment of, **1035–1051**
Direct oral anticoagulants. *See* Anticoagulants.

E

Ecarin clotting time, testing direct oral anticoagulant activity with, 1000
Edoxaban, for atrial fibrillation, 1027
    monitoring effects of, 999–1000
    reversal of, with andexanet alpha, 1091–1093
Elderly patients, over 75, use of direct oral anticoagulants in, 1058–1062
Electronic health records, meaningful use of, 1124–1126
Eliquis. *See* Apixaban.
Enoxaparin, trials comparing with oral dosing of apixaban after joint replacement surgery,
    1012–1014

F

Factor IX, role in thrombosis in humans, 1104
Factor IXa inhibitors, clinical trials of, 1105–1106

Factor Xa, testing for inhibition of, in patients on direct oral anticoagulants, 1000–1001
Factor Xa inhibitors, history of, 1010–1011
    pharmacology of, in treatment of VTE, 1036–1037
Factor XI, antisense-induced reduction of levels of, 1107–1108
    role in thrombin generation, 1101
    role in thrombosis in humans, 1104–1105

H

Heart valve replacement, use of dabigatran in patients with mechanical heart valves, 1027–1028
Heath policy, regulatory impact on thrombosis treatment, prevention, and anticoagulant use, **1115–1135**
        electronic health record meaningful use, 1124–1126
        litigation, 1130
        National Action Plan for Adverse Drug Event Prevention, 1126
        organization interactions and performance measures, 1116–1119
        point scoring systems, 1121–1124
            Hospital Acquired Conditions Reduction Program, 1121–1122
            Hospital Consumer Assessment of Healthcare Providers and Systems, 1122–1123
            Value-Based Purchasing, 1124
        postmarketing surveillance, 1126–1129
        product contamination and pharmaceutical supply chain, 1129–1130
        surgical care improvement projects, 1120–1121
        targeted performance standards, 1119–1120
            stroke management standards, 1119–1120
Heparin, discovery of, 988–990
Hip replacement. See Joint replacement surgery.
History, of antithrombotic therapy, **987–993**
        aspirin use as, 991–992
        discovery of heparin, 988–990
        discovery of the vitamin K antagonists, 990
Hospital Acquired Conditions Reduction Program, 1121–1122
Hospital Consumer Assessment of Healthcare Providers and Systems, 1122

I

Idarucizumab, for reversal of oral direct anticoagulants, 1030–1031, 1090–1091
Intrinsic pathway of coagulation, as target for antithrombotic therapy, **1085–1098**
        in models of blood coagulation, 1100–1103
            cascade-waterfall model of thrombin generation, 1100–1101
            kallikrein-kinin system and contact activation, 1103
            tissue factor-initiated thrombin generation and role of Factor XI, 1101
        thrombosis and, 1103–1105
            animal models, 1103–1104
            Factor IX and VIII thrombosis in humans, 1104
            Factor XI thrombosis in humans, 1104–1105
            intrinsic pathway in humans, 1105
            kallikrein-kinin system in humans, 1105
        trials of agents targeting, 1105–1108

Intrinsic (*continued*)
        antisense-induced reduction of Factor XI levels, 1107–1108
        Factor IXa inhibitors, 1105–1106
        targeting the kallikrein-kinin system, 1108

J

Joint replacement surgery, venous thromboembolism prophylaxis after, **1007–1018**
    efficacy of, 1014
    Factor Xa inhibitors, history of, 1010–1011
    safety of, 1014–1015
    summary of trials to prevent DVT and PE, 1011–1014

K

Kallikrein-kinin system, and contact activation, role in thrombin generation, 1103
    role in thrombosis in humans, 1105
    targeting, trials of, 1108
Knee replacement. *See* Joint replacement surgery.

L

Liquid chromatography/tandem mass spectrometry, testing direct oral anticoagulant
    activity with, 1000
Lixiana. *See* Edoxaban.
Low body weight, use of direct oral anticoagulants in patients with, 1054–1058

M

Mechanical heart valves, use of dabigatran in patients with, 1027–1028
Monitoring, for effects of direct oral anticoagulants, **995–1006**
        assessing reversal of, 1003
        diagnostic options, 997–1002
            coagulation testing, 997
            global assays, 1001
            liquid chromatography/tandem mass spectrometry methodology, 1000
            Russell viper venom time, 1001
            screening coagulation tests (PT and aPTT), 997–1000
            testing specific for measurement of direct thrombin inhibitory activity, 1000–1001
        levels of, and clinical outcomes, 1002
        limitations of assays, 1002–1003

N

National Action Plan for Adverse Drug Event Prevention, 1126
Non-vitamin K antagonist oral anticoagulants (NOAC). *See* Anticoagulants, direct oral.
Novel oral anticoagulants (NOACs). *See* Anticoagulants, direct oral.

O

Obese patients, use of direct oral anticoagulants in, 1054–1058
Oral anticoagulants, direct. *See* Anticoagulants.
Outcomes, clinical, assessment of direct oral anticoagulant effects on, 1002

P

Perioperative management, of patients on direct oral anticoagulants, **1073–1084**
    with high thrombotic risk patient, 1076–1077
    in a low bleed risk procedure, 1077–1079
    in a minimal bleed risk procedure, 1074–1076
    in urgent surgery, 1079–1081
Pharmaceuticals. *See also specific drug names.*, litigation related to adverse drug
    events, 1130
    postmarketing surveillance by FDA, 1126–1129
    product contamination and supply chain, 1129–1130
Postmarketing surveillance, by FDA, 1126–1129
Pradaxa. *See* Dabigatran.
Prothrombin time (PT), coagulation testing in patients on direct oral anticoagulants,
    997–1000
        apixaban, 999
        dabigatran, 998
        edoxaban, 999–1000
        rivaroxaban, 998–999
Pulmonary embolism (PE), trials of regulation of coagulation in joint replacement surgery to
    prevent, 1011–1012
    use of direct oral anticoagulants for treatment of, **1035–1051**

R

Regulatory impact, on thrombosis treatment, prevention, and anticoagulant use,
    1115–1135
        electronic health record meaningful use, 1124–1126
        litigation, 1130
        National Action Plan for Adverse Drug Event Prevention, 1126
        organization interactions and performance measures, 1116–1119
        point scoring systems, 1121–1124
            Hospital Acquired Conditions Reduction Program, 1121–1122
            Hospital Consumer Assessment of Healthcare Providers and Systems,
                1122–1123
            Value-Based Purchasing, 1124
        postmarketing surveillance, 1126–1129
        product contamination and pharmaceutical supply chain, 1129–1130
        surgical care improvement projects, 1120–1121
        targeted performance standards, 1119–1120
            stroke management standards, 1119–1120
Renal impairment, use of direct oral anticoagulants in patients with moderate or severe,
    1062–1065
Reversal, of direct oral anticoagulants, assessment of, 1001–1002
Reversal agents, for direct oral anticoagulants, 1030–1031, **1085–1098**
        attributes of, 1086
        current state of, 1088–1090
        future of, 1094
        specific agents for, 1090–1094
            andexanet alpha, 1091–1093
            ciraparantag, 1093–1094

Reversal (*continued*)
  idarucizumab, 1090–1091
  for vitamin K antagonists, 1086–1088
  when are they needed, 1086
Rivaroxaban, for atrial fibrillation, 1023–1026
  monitoring effects of, 998–999
  reversal of, with andexanet alpha, 1091–1093
Russell viper venom time, testing direct oral anticoagulant activity with, 1001

S

Savaysa. *See* Edoxaban.
Stroke management standards, 1119–1120
Surgery, perioperative management of patients on direct oral anticoagulants, **1073–1084**
  with high thrombotic risk patient, 1076–1077
  in a low bleed risk procedure, 1077–1079
  in a minimal bleed risk procedure, 1074–1076
  in urgent surgery, 1079–1081
Surgical Care Improvement Project, 1120–1121

T

Thrombin clotting time, testing direct oral anticoagulant activity with, 1000
Thrombophilia, use of direct oral anticoagulants in patients with, 1066–1067
Thrombosis, intrinsic pathway and, 1103–1105
  animal models, 1103–1104
  Factor IX and VIII thrombosis in humans, 1104
  Factor XI thrombosis in humans, 1104–1105
  intrinsic pathway in humans, 1105
  kallikrein-kinin system in humans, 1105
Total hip arthroplasty. *See* Joint replacement surgery.
Total knee arthroplasty. *See* Joint replacement surgery.
Trough levels, in coagulation testing in patients on direct oral anticoagulants, **995–1006**

V

Value-Based Purchasing program, 1124
Venous thromboembolism (VTE), prophylaxis after joint replacement surgery, **1007–1018**
  efficacy of, 1014
  Factor Xa inhibitors, history of, 1010–1011
  safety of, 1014–1015
  summary of trials to prevent DVT and PE, 1011–1014
  use of direct oral anticoagulants for treatment of, **1035–1051**
    for acute phase of treatment, 1038–1039
    for extended treatment, 1039–1041
    pharmacologic properties of, 1036–1037
    in routine clinical practice, 1046
    in special populations, 1041–1046
    summary of evidence, 1046–1047
Vitamin K antagonists, discovery of, 990
  reversal agent for, 1086–1088

W

Warfarin, efficacy, safety and limitations for patients with atrial fibrillation, 1021–1022

X

Xarelto. *See* Rivaroxaban.

UNITED STATES POSTAL SERVICE®
Statement of Ownership, Management, and Circulation
(All Periodicals Publications Except Requester Publications)

1. Publication Title	2. Publication Number	3. Filing Date
HEMATOLOGY/ONCOLOGY CLINICS OF NORTH AMERICA	002 - 473	9/18/2016

4. Issue Frequency	5. Number of Issues Published Annually	6. Annual Subscription Price
FEB, APR, JUN, AUG, OCT, DEC	6	$385.00

7. Complete Mailing Address of Known Office of Publication (Not printer) (Street, city, county, state, and ZIP+4®)

ELSEVIER INC.
360 PARK AVENUE SOUTH
NEW YORK, NY 10010-1710

Contact Person
STEPHEN R. BUSHING
Telephone (Include area code)
215-239-3688

8. Complete Mailing Address of Headquarters or General Business Office of Publisher (Not printer)

ELSEVIER INC.
360 PARK AVENUE SOUTH
NEW YORK, NY 10010-1710

9. Full Names and Complete Mailing Addresses of Publisher, Editor, and Managing Editor (Do not leave blank)

Publisher (Name and complete mailing address)

ADRIANNE BRIGIDO, ELSEVIER INC.
1600 JOHN F KENNEDY BLVD. SUITE 1800
PHILADELPHIA, PA 19103-2899

Editor (Name and complete mailing address)

JENNIFER FLYNN-BRIGGS, ELSEVIER INC.
1600 JOHN F KENNEDY BLVD. SUITE 1800
PHILADELPHIA, PA 19103-2899

Managing Editor (Name and complete mailing address)

PATRICK MANLEY, ELSEVIER INC.
1600 JOHN F KENNEDY BLVD. SUITE 1800
PHILADELPHIA, PA 19103-2899

10. Owner (Do not leave blank. If the publication is owned by a corporation, give the name and address of the corporation immediately followed by the names and addresses of all stockholders owning or holding 1 percent or more of the total amount of stock. If not owned by a corporation, give the names and addresses of the individual owners. If owned by a partnership or other unincorporated firm, give its name and address as well as those of each individual owner. If the publication is published by a nonprofit organization, give its name and address.)

Full Name	Complete Mailing Address
WHOLLY OWNED SUBSIDIARY OF REED/ELSEVIER, US HOLDINGS	1600 JOHN F KENNEDY BLVD. SUITE 1800 PHILADELPHIA, PA 19103-2899

11. Known Bondholders, Mortgagees, and Other Security Holders Owning or Holding 1 Percent or More of Total Amount of Bonds, Mortgages, or Other Securities. If none, check box ▶ ☐ None

Full Name	Complete Mailing Address
N/A	

12. Tax Status (For completion by nonprofit organizations authorized to mail at nonprofit rates) (Check one)
The purpose, function, and nonprofit status of this organization and the exempt status for federal income tax purposes:
☐ Has Not Changed During Preceding 12 Months
☐ Has Changed During Preceding 12 Months (Publisher must submit explanation of change with this statement)

13. Publication Title	14. Issue Date for Circulation Data Below
HEMATOLOGY/ONCOLOGY CLINICS OF NORTH AMERICA	AUGUST 2016

PS Form 3526, July 2014 [Page 1 of 4 (see instructions page 4)] PSN: 7530-01-000-9931 PRIVACY NOTICE: See our privacy policy on www.usps.com.

---

15. Extent and Nature of Circulation		Average No. Copies Each Issue During Preceding 12 Months	No. Copies of Single Issue Published Nearest to Filing Date
a. Total Number of Copies (Net press run)		371	474
b. Paid Circulation (By Mail and Outside the Mail)	(1) Mailed Outside-County Paid Subscriptions Stated on PS Form 3541 (Include paid distribution above nominal rate, advertiser's proof copies, and exchange copies)	93	132
	(2) Mailed In-County Paid Subscriptions Stated on PS Form 3541 (Include paid distribution above nominal rate, advertiser's proof copies, and exchange copies)	0	0
	(3) Paid Distribution Outside the Mails Including Sales Through Dealers and Carriers, Street Vendors, Counter Sales, and Other Paid Distribution Outside USPS®	63	90
	(4) Paid Distribution by Other Classes of Mail Through the USPS (e.g. First-Class Mail®)	0	0
c. Total Paid Distribution (Sum of 15b (1), (2), (3), and (4)) ▶		156	222
d. Free or Nominal Rate Distribution (By Mail and Outside the Mail)	(1) Free or Nominal Rate Outside-County Copies included on PS Form 3541	78	122
	(2) Free or Nominal Rate In-County Copies Included on PS Form 3541	0	0
	(3) Free or Nominal Rate Copies Mailed at Other Classes Through the USPS (e.g. First-Class Mail)	0	0
	(4) Free or Nominal Rate Distribution Outside the Mail (Carriers or other means)	0	0
e. Total Free or Nominal Rate Distribution (Sum of 15d (1), (2), (3) and (4)) ▶		78	122
f. Total Distribution (Sum of 15c and 15e) ▶		234	344
g. Copies not Distributed (See Instructions to Publishers #4 (page #3)) ▶		137	130
h. Total (Sum of 15f and g) ▶		371	474
i. Percent Paid (15c divided by 15f times 100) ▶		67%	64%

PS Form 3526, July 2014 (Page 2 of 4)

16. Electronic Copy Circulation	Average No. Copies Each Issue During Preceding 12 Months	No. Copies of Single Issue Published Nearest to Filing Date
a. Paid Electronic Copies ▶	0	0
b. Total Paid Print Copies (Line 15c) + Paid Electronic Copies (Line 16a) ▶	156	222
c. Total Print Distribution (Line 15f) + Paid Electronic Copies (Line 16a) ▶	234	344
d. Percent Paid (Both Print & Electronic Copies) (16b divided by 16c × 100) ▶	67%	64%

☒ I certify that 50% of all my distributed copies (electronic and print) are paid above a nominal price.

17. Publication of Statement of Ownership
☒ If the publication is a general publication, publication of this statement is required. Will be printed in the OCTOBER 2016 issue of this publication. ☐ Publication not required.

18. Signature and Title of Editor, Publisher, Business Manager, or Owner

Stephen R. Bushing Date 9/18/2016

STEPHEN R. BUSHING - INVENTORY DISTRIBUTION CONTROL MANAGER

I certify that all information furnished on this form is true and complete. I understand that anyone who furnishes false or misleading information on this form or who omits material or information requested on the form may be subject to criminal sanctions (including fines and imprisonment) and/or civil sanctions (including civil penalties).

PS Form 3526, July 2014 (Page 3 of 4) PRIVACY NOTICE: See our privacy policy on www.usps.com.

Moving?

Make sure your subscription moves with you!

To notify us of your new address, find your **Clinics Account Number** (located on your mailing label above your name), and contact customer service at:

Email: journalscustomerservice-usa@elsevier.com

800-654-2452 (subscribers in the U.S. & Canada)
314-447-8871 (subscribers outside of the U.S. & Canada)

Fax number: 314-447-8029

Elsevier Health Sciences Division
Subscription Customer Service
3251 Riverport Lane
Maryland Heights, MO 63043

*To ensure uninterrupted delivery of your subscription,
please notify us at least 4 weeks in advance of move.

Printed and bound by CPI Group (UK) Ltd, Croydon, CR0 4YY

12/10/2024

01773485-0003